# wake up to
# YOGA

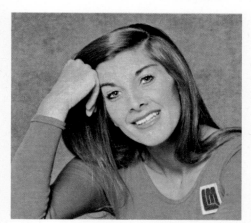

## Lyn Marshall

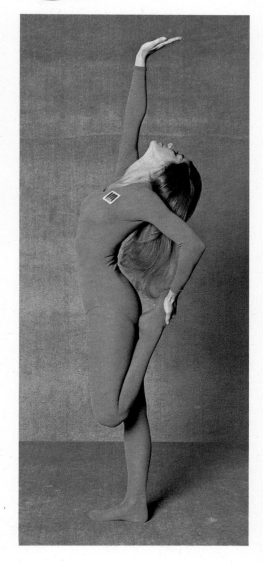

*Listen to your body*
*Handle it with care*
*Step inside it with your mind*
*And then you're almost there!*
                        *L.M.*

WARD LOCK LIMITED LONDON

© Yoga World Limited 1975

ISBN 0 7063 5077 4

First published in 1975 in Great Britain by
Ward Lock Limited, 47 Marylebone Lane,
London W1M 6AX a Pentos Company

Six Impressions 1975
Two Impressions 1976
Three Impressions 1977
Reprinted 1978, 1979, 1981

Photographs by Simon Farrell;
LWT/Yoga World Limited.
Designed by Andrew Shoolbred

Printed in Great Britain by Optima Print and Packaging Ltd.
Bound by Pitman Press, Bath

# Contents

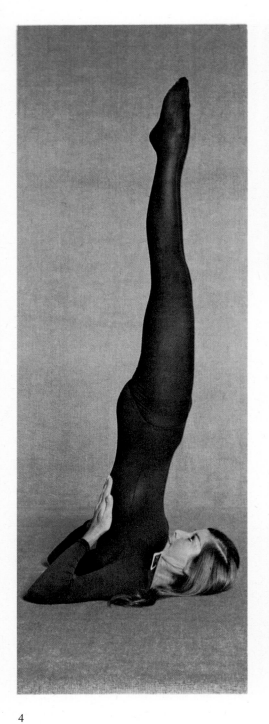

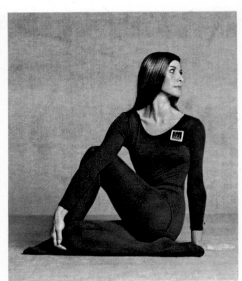

Full Twist

Completed Shoulder Stand

Completed Leg Pull

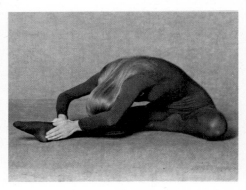

4

# Introduction

If anyone had mentioned the word **Yoga** to me a few years ago, it would immediately have conjured up images of weird men tied up in knots, meditating in the foothills of the Himalayas. I am sure that there are many people who still think this way, but nothing could be further from the truth. It is a fact that Yoga is ancient and originated in the East, but there is no reason why we cannot adapt it and benefit from it here in modern-day Western society, and that is what *Wake up to Yoga* is all about.

## Biography

I was originally trained to be a classical ballet dancer, and on completion of my training, I went to Italy to join an operatic company and I lived and worked there happily for five years.

During the latter part of my stay in Italy I found that I was being offered more and more modelling work, and I discovered that not only was this effortless compared to dancing, but it was also a much more lucrative occupation. On my return to this country, I became a full-time model, and though I was successful and made a lot of money, I found I was getting very little satisfaction. Then in 1970 I was introduced to Yoga and my whole life changed.

At first I did only one or two of the movements a day, simply because it felt good, but the more I got out of them the longer I wanted to spend each day practising, and the hungrier I became for knowledge about Yoga.

I felt marvellous and I wanted to know why.

I began to study, and subsequently went on to research the medical angle with an Indian doctor who had both studied and practised the Yoga movements for fifteen years. I realized that not only had I found the most medically sound and logical way of keeping my body in peak condition, but having experienced various other forms of exercize and keep-fit as well as a rigorous ballet training, I was convinced that this was definitely the easiest and the most pleasurable way.

There were no energetic or repetitive movements such as I had been used to, no feelings of exhaustion and fatigue. In fact, quite the reverse. I felt refreshed, relaxed and revitalized afterwards.

My friends, noticing the marked physical and psychological change in me, were constantly asking me to teach them the movements. This I eventually did, and seeing them benefit as I had, convinced me that I wanted to teach and pass on what I had learned so that many others could benefit as well.

A short while after this my Yoga school was born, and I knew then that this was what I wanted to do with my life. At my school I get immense satisfaction watching my students enrich their lives with Yoga, and now I hope that through my television series, record and book many of you will begin to practise and receive the tremendous benefits that Yoga has to offer.

## What is Yoga?

Physical or Hatha Yoga is a series of extremely well thought-out postures or positions that move and improve virtually every part of the human body.

They are not exercizes, but if you practise the Yoga movements regularly, it is easy to reach peak physical condition, spending very little time and a minimum of effort. This is quite the reverse of the normal rigorous activities that one expects to have to undertake to improve one's body and health.

There are lots of self-improvement gadgets on the market as well as numerous services, all claiming that they will **do it for you**. Well, although some of these might work for a period of time, the effect can only be temporary. Permanent body improvement must come from inside your own body. It must be a natural body movement, and Yoga done my way is not only natural it is also very enjoyable. What is more, its effectiveness can be felt as soon as you start to practise.

**In short—it works.**

## My method

My method of Yoga is first and foremost very pleasurable to do. It is not a physical work-out of any sort, but a series of gentle stretches that when put together become the Yoga movements.

You need spend only a few short minutes a day practising to feel the enormous benefits that Yoga done my way will bring. However, like most things in life that one enjoys, it is something that you will probably want to devote more and more time to. Add to that the fact that you will both look and feel marvellous, and you will know that you are on to a good thing.

There are various forms of physical or Hatha Yoga being practised today. Many of them place great emphasis on attaining the finished positions or postures, and this unfortunately has caused many would-be students to drop out. They find it either too much of a strain to get into these positions, or, as many are unable to get anywhere near achieving the positions. they feel that continuing would be totally pointless.

With my method of Yoga, there is no finished position that one **has** to attain. Emphasis is placed on moving slowly and smoothly, and the amount of stretching that you do to begin with is so slight as to be hardly noticeable. You stop as soon as you reach your own body's natural and comfortable limit, and it is by holding this position still for a set count, that you establish the stretch in the body and limbs. Each time you come to repeat the movement you are then able to go a little further. This way the body progresses at its own speed and you never experience any strain.

My Yoga is for everyone, young, old, fat or thin, in whatever physical condition. From the very first time that you execute a movement you will be receiving benefit, no matter what stage of the position you are in, as long as you go to your own comfortable limit.

It is partly for this reason that my Yoga movements are done in extreme slow motion. If you move slowly, you are aware of your body and can feel exactly when you have gone far enough—and you stop. Moving quickly you know you have gone too far only when it is too late, and the muscles or ligaments are pulled and the damage is done.

My teaching is very westernized, and I do not therefore believe in using eastern terminology, as this can be very confusing. All of my movements and postures have easily identifiable English names, which will quickly become familiar to you.

I believe that one Yoga movement executed my way is of more value than ten normal exercizes, and for this reason seldom is any movement performed more than twice. The normal repetitive 1-2, 1-2 type exercizes can not only become monotonous, but they also tend to overactivate the heart, putting a strain on it, to increase the appetite, to cause perspiration and a feeling of exhaustion—and usually a sense of relief when it is all over.

My Yoga movements, on the other hand, leave you feeling refreshed, relaxed, invigorated and revitalized—even if you spend just a few minutes doing them.

## How to use Yoga

Yoga can be **used**, and I really do mean used in the fullest sense of the word, to improve your daily life, no matter who you are or what you do.

You do not necessarily have to be looking for a spiritually uplifting experience, or indeed involvement of any kind. You can simply use the movements to achieve any or all of the following:

Lose weight—either generally or in specific areas of the body.

Learn how to relax properly.

Rid yourself of back problems.

Remove mental strain and tension.

Improve your figure.

Strengthen and recondition your entire body.

Stay relaxed under pressure.

Improve your concentration.

Become more sensually aware of yourself and others.

Improve your circulation and breathing.

Get relief from conditions such as insomnia, headaches, migraine, sinusitis and asthma.

Improve the condition of your skin, your eyes and your hair. (Yes, there is even a movement that stimulates the blood flow to the hair follicles, promoting hair growth.)

Improve your balance and posture.

Regain agility and youth.

You can use the Yoga movements for all of these things and many many more, far too numerous to mention. If you feel this claim seems somewhat exaggerated, then I urge you to practise the appropriate movements—the results will be all the proof you need.

My style of Yoga is designed for people who lead normal lives—doing normal things, so that it can be used in a practical way to fit in with your life.

## What do you need?

You need only the floor space to do the movements, preferably privacy, so that you can relax completely and concentrate on what you are doing, and a few minutes in which to practise the movements. This will be no hardship, because once you see how effective the movements are you will find your Yoga practice becoming a valuable part of your everyday life.

## Does Yoga change your life?

You do not have to alter your life one bit to practise Yoga, but changes will occur. The first and most obvious change is that you will both look and feel better. Also, the more you practise, the more you will find subtle little changes taking place. For example, you tend to slow down and relax more when eating, and many people tell me that they suddenly realize that they are satisfied with far less food than they were previously used to.

Sensitivity and awareness increase, and you may find that your taste buds become more alive and you go off certain foods, developing preferences for others. This is not something that you make yourself do, it just seems to happen over a period of time. Likewise, a lot of students tell me that they have cut down on their smoking without consciously setting out to do so. The nice thing about these changes is that invariably they are for the better. Who, after all, wants to continue to smoke heavily with the threat of lung cancer hanging over them? Moreover, there is never a feeling of deprivation, since you do not set out to bring about these changes—they just happen naturally.

You will also find that your concentration improves and your mental alertness too, and as you practise your self-confidence will grow and you will become more self-assured.

## Stiffness and age

You are never too young or too old to do Yoga. I have students ranging in age from eight to over eighty. What you must remember is that it is not important how stiff or out of condition you think you are, or how well you are able to do these movements at first. The gentleness of the movements makes them ideal for both the elderly and the acutely stiff.

If you execute them carefully, without straining or trying to go too far, you will quickly see a marked improvement, as your body stretches a little more each time you perform the movements.

It has been my experience that the Yoga movements have been particularly beneficial where chronic stiffening of the joints has occurred, as in osteoarthritis, and a great degree of success can be achieved through regular and gentle practice of the movements.

## Not straining

**You must never experience any strain while performing the Yoga movements.** Go only as far as is comfortable for you in all of the positions, taking your body to its **own natural limit**. It is the holding of that position absolutely still for the required count that will ensure that each time you repeat that movement you will be able to go a little further. Trying to do too much too quickly will not only cause strain but will actually retard your progress.

The holding count for most of the positions is five. Count to yourself at approximately the same speed as seconds. Where the count differs, you will find it clearly indicated in my instructions.

When you begin to practise, you may find that although a position may have been comfortable to start with, during the holding period it becomes increasingly uncomfortable. Should this happen, come out of the position—as instructed—immediately. In a very short space of time you will be able to maintain your position for the full count.

## Competition

There is no such thing as competition in Yoga. Every **body** is different. It does not matter that one person can get into a seemingly advanced position in a week of practice, while another is still in a comparatively elementary position after practising for nearly a year. As long as you go to your own comfortable limit you are getting the same benefit, no matter what stage of the position you are in. Likewise, it does not follow that someone who is slim and athletic will progress any faster than a middle-aged person who is of heavy build, so be aware only of yourself. There is no hurry, and no prize for the person who reaches a certain position first. You are receiving full benefit from your first day of practice, because you are listening to your body, and allowing it to take you a little further only when it is ready.

## Slow motion

Everything is done in extreme slow motion and with control, really feeling what is happening to the body. The reason for this is twofold. Firstly, if you are moving slowly, you can feel exactly when you have gone far enough—and you stop. This prevents any pulling or straining of the muscles, ligaments and joints. Secondly, you are concentrating and becoming so aware of the particular section of the body that you are moving, that automatically all other thoughts are erased from your mind. This clearance of the mind, even if it is only for a few short minutes, brings about tremendous mental relaxation.

You may find that moving slowly is a little difficult at first because we are so used to doing everything quickly, but as you practise and become more aware of your body, you will find yourself slowing down.

## Allowing your body to unwind

As well as executing the movements and postures correctly, it is also very important that you allow your body to unwind at its own natural pace after performing a movement. So whether you are continuing with another movement or returning to the day's activities, take care to spend at least a few moments in the relaxation positions, where indicated, following specific movements.

## Breathing

Breathing should be executed slowly and deeply through the nose while doing the Yoga movements.

Once you know the movements, you can follow the breathing instructions in the back of the book, but do not try to learn the breathing at the same time as the movements, as this can only result in confusion.

Learning and executing the movements correctly should be your first priority, just breathing normally through the nose. When you are absolutely sure that you know the movements, begin to use the individual breathing instructions as set out on pages 91-95.

You may find at first that you cannot hold your breath for the required count as instructed. Do not worry. This takes a little practice, and in time you will find that you can retain the breath for longer and longer periods. If you run out of breath during a movement—take another.

## Practice—when, where and how?

Practise any of the movements whenever you have the time and space. Preferably somewhere quiet where you won't be disturbed. You can do just one or as many of the postures as you wish. If you would like to go through a routine of the postures, then ideally you should begin and end your session with a few minutes in the Corpse posture (the position of deep relaxation).

Never try to do as many movements as you can when practising—you will probably rush them and get very little benefit. Slowness and smoothness is the key, and it is far better to spend ten minutes doing one posture correctly than four or five hurriedly.

Try to have as little food in the stomach as possible, especially if you are planning on going through a routine of postures (preferably no food for an hour and a half before your practice session).

It can be tremendously beneficial to use certain of the movements during your working day, and in many cases your lunch hour is the only break you get; so eat after your few minutes of Yoga rather than before.

Practise by following my instructions very carefully. Step by step they will take you right through the movements and into the relaxation positions that follow. In a short while you will get to know the movements off by heart and can just refer to the photographs to check that you are doing them correctly.

## Practice clothes

You should be able to move the body in any direction, allowing it complete freedom. The breathing apparatus needs to be able to work efficiently, so ideally nothing tight or restricting should be worn around the waist.

For women a leotard and tights are best, and for men trousers or loose pants with an elasticated waistband. A track suit, for example, would be fine.

Obviously, if you are going to practise the movements at work, then a complete change of clothes is rarely possible or practical. So just make sure that you loosen your clothing as much as you can around the waist, and take off your shoes when appropriate.

## Yoga Practice Mats

Floor surfaces vary a great deal, and if you are going to practise regularly then it is worth investing in a Yoga practice mat. These are specially designed so that they are not only firm enough to support you and allow

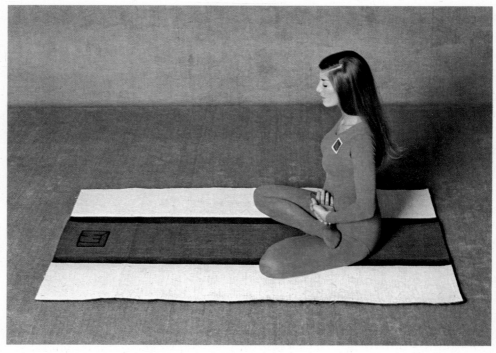

you to balance properly, but have sufficient give to cushion your bones and joints in some of the sitting, kneeling and lying postures.

These mats can be packed away and kept clean between your practice sessions, and can be used indoors or out.

## Check with your doctor

Though it is clear that Yoga improves your health and can also be very therapeutic in eliminating many physical ailments and disorders, **it must never be used as a substitute for medical treatment.**

If you are ill or have a history of serious illness, check with your doctor before you begin to practise. He knows your medical history and is therefore qualified to tell you whether you can safely undertake these movements.

Many doctors are now realizing the benefits and advantages that Yoga has to offer, and as well as having doctors among my students I am finding that more and more doctors are referring patients to me. The extreme gentleness of this form of Yoga, makes it the ideal system of body movement for patients who must not or cannot undertake strenuous exercizes.

## Points to remember

1 Although the Yoga movements are easy and pleasurable to do, you must approach them in a serious manner if you are to get maximum benefit out of them.

2 Read the instructions relating to each movement or posture and study the pictures carefully before you attempt to perform it.

3 Whether you practise for three or thirty minutes, devote all your attention to what you are doing, and try to concentrate completely on whichever part of the body is being used.

4 Remember to do **everything** slowly and smoothly. This rule applies not only when doing the actual postures, but also when you lie down or get up before and after a movement. Don't rush—do it slowly.

5 Take care to position the body exactly as directed, and even though the placement of fingers, elbows, chin etc. may seem trivial, this is of infinite importance to the movements.

13

# 1 Relaxation

Most people find complete relaxation a difficult thing to achieve. You can't force yourself to relax no matter how hard you try—it just doesn't work. You have to **allow** yourself to relax by letting go of every single muscle in the body and the face, and then clearing the mind.

The lives we lead today are more hectic than ever before, and the stresses, strains and tensions that are part of our lives will take their toll, and inevitably our bodies and minds will suffer. It is vital, therefore, to give the mind and body time-out to relax completely, if we are to maintain both in good working order.

The ability to relax completely at will, both physically and mentally, is something that only few people can do, but as you will see this can be achieved easily once you know how. It simply entails lying down on the floor for a few minutes in the Corpse posture.

## The Corpse

The Corpse, or posture of deep relaxation, is a position in which every muscle in the face and body is allowed to be completely at rest, and in time also the mind. Blood can flow freely throughout the body and head refreshing them, while the breathing apparatus is not restricted in any way and can therefore function at maximum efficiency.

The benefits of lying in this Corpse position relaxing for just a few minutes will be felt immediately. Tiredness and fatigue will disappear. Nervous tension and anxiety will go. Feelings of depression and irritability fade away and you are left feeling refreshed, relaxed and invigorated.

Also, you will have relaxed deeply and completely, and though it may only have been for a few minutes, that is sufficient time to have recharged your entire organism, so that you will discover a new source of physical and mental energy enabling you to cope with far more than you could previously handle.

Don't let your surroundings inhibit you. You need only floor space and the privacy, so whether you are in the middle of the housework or at the office—maybe in your lunch hour—take a few minutes to lie down on the floor and see how good it feels.

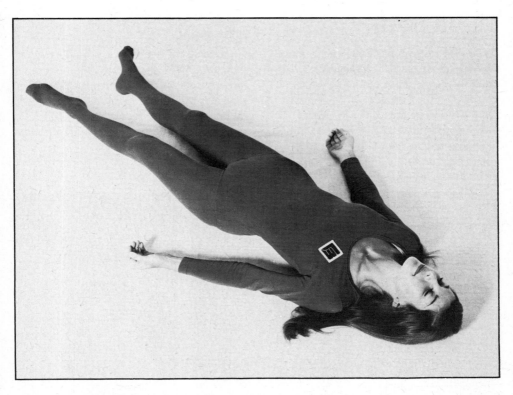

1 Lie down slowly flat on your back with legs together and arms at your sides.

2 Allow the feet to fall gently open, relaxing all the leg and feet muscles.

3 Put the hands palms upwards a few inches away from the body, and let your fingers curl if they want to. Let your arms go limp.

4 Tilt the head back a couple of inches by raising your chin, and close your eyes.

5 Let go of all of the facial muscles, and if your mouth wants to drop open—let it.

6 Slow the breathing down by inhaling deeply, and then exhaling as slowly as you can and not taking another breath until you absolutely have to.

7 Concentrate completely on your breathing, and don't let your attention wander.

8 Stay in the position for as long as you like, but take great care to get up slowly.

**Note**
Whenever you execute a movement that begins by lying down flat on the back, always adopt the Corpse posture for a few moments to relax the body before you start and again at the end of the movement.

The Corpse is the ideal position for sleep, and the use of pillows will not affect the deep relaxation that this position affords.

15

# The Refresher

This is one of the most gentle yet effective movements you can do, and it makes it an ideal first movement to try, either on its own or after the Corpse.

It is simply relaxing the body over, allowing just the weight of the head, arms and hands to take your body as far as it will go comfortably, holding for a count of ten and straightening up slowly.

It relaxes the head, neck, shoulders, arms, hands and back, and gently stretches the lower back and backs of the legs. Blood can flow into the head, and this has a tremendously refreshing effect.

Remember to move slowly and smoothly at all times.

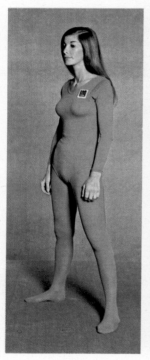 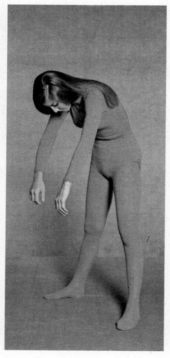 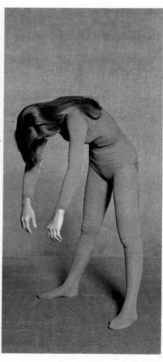

1  Stand straight with the legs and feet eighteen to twenty inches apart, and your arms at your sides.

2  Allow the body to relax forward, gently letting the head, hands and arms just hang.

3  In time the body will come over a little further.

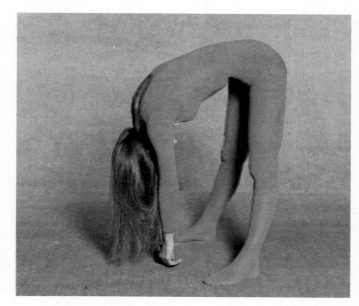

4 Eventually, without pushing or straining, the body will come right over from the hips like this.

Hold the position absolutely still for a count of ten.

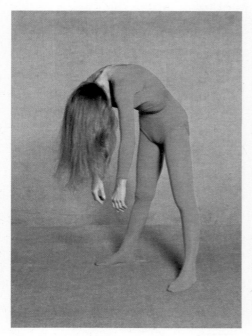

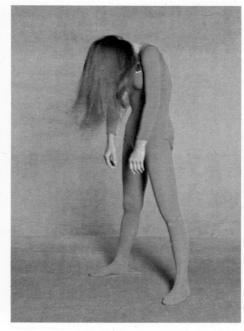

5 Slowly straighten up, letting your head, hands and arms stay relaxed.

6 Straighten your back, bringing your head up last.

# 2 Tension

Tension is something that we have all experienced at some time or another, and it can manifest itself in all sorts of ways. We can become physically run down; prone to headaches and stomach upsets; become easily fatigued, and either over- or under-eat. We also tend to get short-tempered, nervous and irritable when we are tense, and fly off the handle for the least little thing. Our brain too becomes less efficient and unable to cope with normal day-to-day problems, causing us to act impulsively rather than rationally.

There are varying degrees of tension, but they all have a detrimental effect on both mind and body. By executing these movements regularly, you will eliminate that tension and also the symptoms that go with it.

One usually feels tension most acutely in the neck area, and at the top of the back between the shoulder blades, and so these movements have been specifically designed to work this stiffness out gently and effectively.

The movements need be performed only once or twice, and can be used wherever you are and as often as you like during the day when you feel the need to relieve that tension. People involved in occupations that cause them to be continually bent over or under pressure, will find these movements immediately effective if performed during their working day.

## Tension Release

This movement is like an internal massage, working out the stiffness and tension from the top of the back, where all the nerve endings meet up and where we feel that awful tightness between the shoulder blades.

When you come to do it, do not become despondent if you cannot join your hands up behind you, let alone get your elbows straight. This is one of the stiffest areas of the body, which is proof in itself that we need to introduce movement into it. Be content at first just to go through the motions of attaining the **lock** (see picture 9) and do not attempt to raise the arms.

Once you can comfortably attain this lock, you can begin to raise the arms, but no more than a few inches at first.

The raising of the arms intensifies the stretch at the top of the spine.

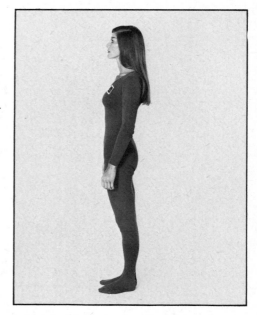

1 Stand with the back straight, head erect and the feet together. Arms at your sides.

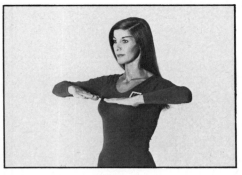

2 Bend the elbows and bring the hands in level with the chest.

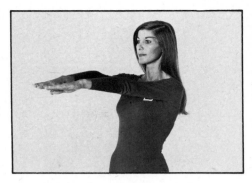

3 Extend the arms straight out in front.

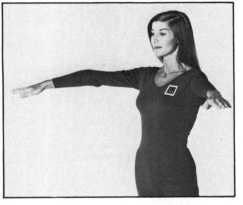

4 Bring the arms around slowly at shoulder level.

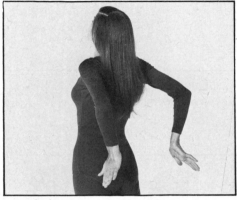

5 Push the chest out and bring the arms down behind the back, bending the elbows and bringing the hands together.

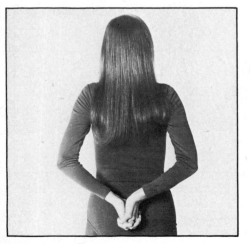

6 Interlock the fingers and press the palms tightly together.

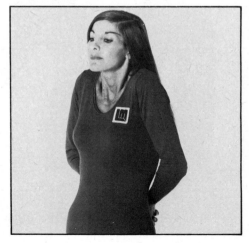

7 Make an exaggerated movement, rotating the shoulders forward and up towards the ears

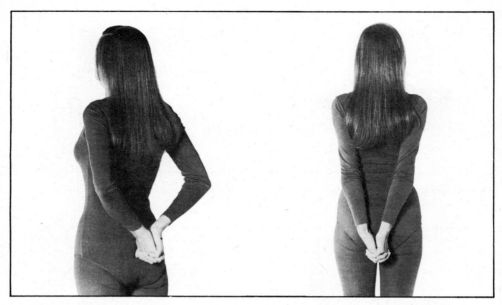

8  Shoulders go back, and as you pull them down try to straighten the elbows.

9  The **lock** is now formed on the top of the spine.

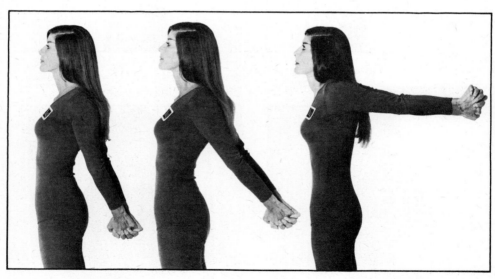

10  Keeping your elbows straight and your hands together, raise the arms only a very moderate distance, keeping the trunk absolutely still.

11  After practising for a while you will be able to raise the arms a little higher.

12  Eventually your arms will be parallel with your shoulders.

Count five, holding the position absolutely still.

20

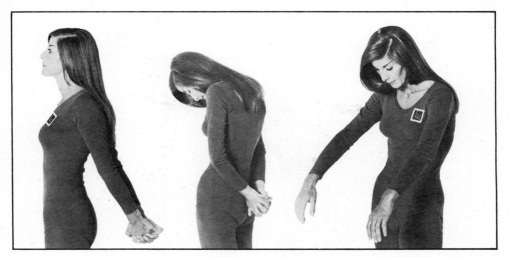

13 Slowly lower the arms, keeping the elbows straight and the hands tightly together.

14 Keep the hands together, but allow the elbows to bend so that the shoulders can come forward to release the lock on the back—and let the head relax forward.

15 Bring the hands and the arms round to the front.

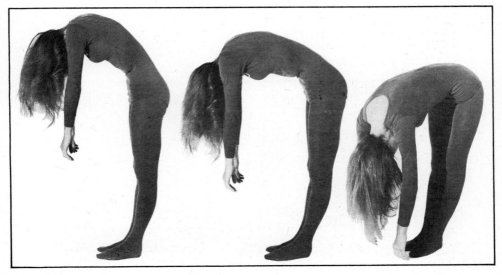

16 Relax the body over and stay like that for a few seconds to let the back unwind, then straighten up slowly.

17 Only relax over as far as you are able.

In time, as the body stretches, you will find you are able to come over further.

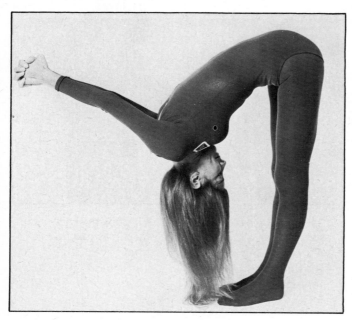

18 This variation is not only working out
the stiffness at the top of the spine, but also
stretching the hamstring muscles at the
backs of the legs. The inversion of the head is
allowing fresh blood into it, to refresh it.

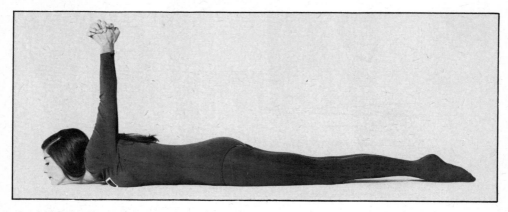

19 This variation is crafty, because when
the arms are raised the body has a tendency
to stoop forward. Lying flat on the stomach,
this is not possible—the floor is in the way.

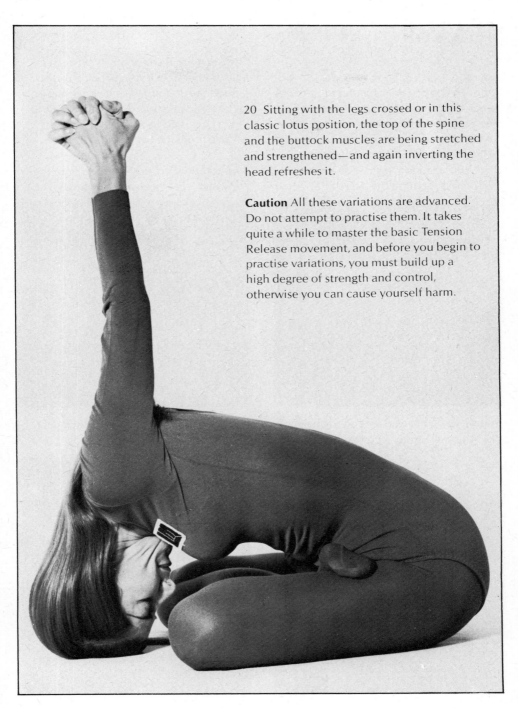

20  Sitting with the legs crossed or in this classic lotus position, the top of the spine and the buttock muscles are being stretched and strengthened—and again inverting the head refreshes it.

**Caution** All these variations are advanced. Do not attempt to practise them. It takes quite a while to master the basic Tension Release movement, and before you begin to practise variations, you must build up a high degree of strength and control, otherwise you can cause yourself harm.

# Neck Roll

This works out the stiffness in the neck, and is also extremely relaxing to do. Although you can do it standing, it is more comfortable to sit, either on a chair or cross-legged on the floor.

Make sure your back is straight, and roll the head gently round, stopping for a couple of seconds in each of the four positions to establish the stretch.

The weight of the head itself will take it over as far as it can go, so don't push it.

Take care to follow the instructions with pictures 4, 5 and 6, as this portion of the movement is designed to work out the stiffness from the back of the neck.

Start by bringing the chin down onto the chest and relax the head completely.

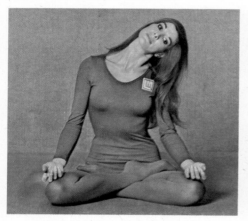

1  Slowly roll the head around to the left. Hold the position for a couple of seconds.

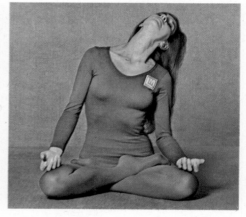

2  Roll the head around to the back— again hold for a couple of seconds.

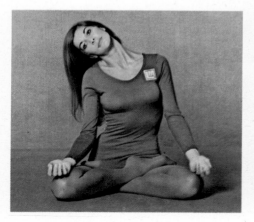

3  Roll the head around to the right and hold again for a couple of seconds.

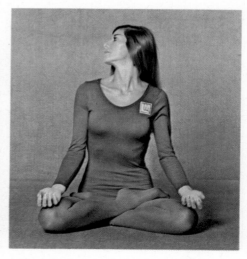

4  Turn the face completely to the right with the chin raised.

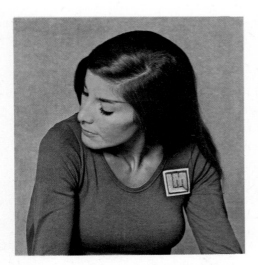

5 Get the chin down onto the chest.

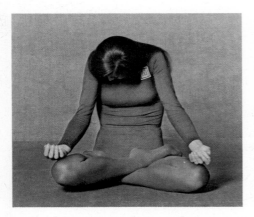

6 Gently push the head down as you slowly bring it round to the front.

Repeat the movement twice in each direction. Once you know the movement— close your eyes.

It has a tremendously calming effect, so if you have time after you have performed the movement keep your head relaxed forward and your eyes closed, relax your face and just stay like that quietly for a few moments.

**Note**
**Do not** attempt the Lotus position as shown. It takes some time before this position can be attained comfortably— so just sit with the legs simply crossed.

# 3  Back Problems

It is amazing how many people suffer from what they loosely describe as 'back trouble'. What is even more amazing is how people seem to accept that aches, pains and stiffness of the back are facts of life that just happen and have to be lived with. Well, they don't just happen. Aches, pains and misplacements of the joints—unless there is a valid medical reason—can occur simply because of lack of movement.

The back, like all the other parts of the body, must be kept mobile and supple if you are to ward off 'back problems'. If you don't keep the back flexible it stiffens up. This means that the joints themselves stiffen up, and it is this stiffness that makes the joints vulnerable to dislocation, slipped discs etc. The back must be supple and strong enough to sustain sudden movements. If it is not, that is when the injuries can occur.

## The Fish

This is an ideal movement to start with, as it gently arches the spine.

Be content to come up only a few inches at first (see picture 2). The head tilted back causes blood to flow in and out and if you perform the movement with your eyes open you may go dizzy. So before you attempt it, read the instructions and study the photographs a few times—see if you can memorize them, and then try to do the movement with your eyes closed.

Go into the Corpse position for a few seconds before you start, so that the body can relax completely.

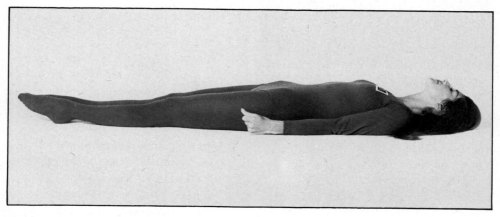

1  Bring the legs and feet together and make fists out of the hands with the thumbs uppermost. Close your eyes.

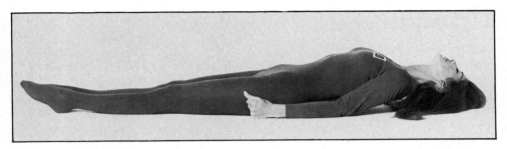

2 Push down hard with your elbows and your fists and arch your spine by pushing the chest up, tilting the head back a little.

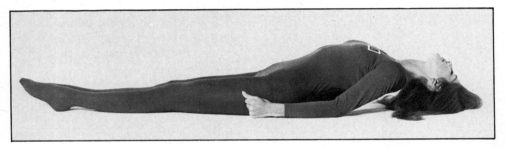

3 After a little practice you will be able to raise a little higher.

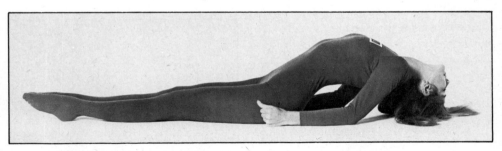

4 Eventually you will be able to achieve a high arch like this.

Count five in your comfortable position—holding still, and then slowly let your head slide back. Allow your back to sink down slowly—don't rush. When you can feel your back flat on the floor again, keep your eyes closed, allow your feet to fall open and let the hands relax onto the backs. Stay like that for a few seconds before repeating the movement.

# Backward Bend

The Backward Bend movement is a progression from the Fish. After practising the Fish for a while, and after your back has started to strengthen, carefully begin to practise the Backward Bend.

Be very precise about the positioning of the body with this movement, as once you have begun you cannot readjust your weight.

It is extremely important that the back is given maximum support, and the hands should be placed directly underneath the shoulders (see picture 4).

You may find that it is uncomfortable to sit on your heels at first (see picture 1), and if this is the case do not attempt the movement just yet. Practise sitting on the heels for a few moments at a time until it becomes more comfortable, and then try the posture.

As well as arching the spine and gaining flexibility, you are strengthening the neck muscles, the shoulders and the back.

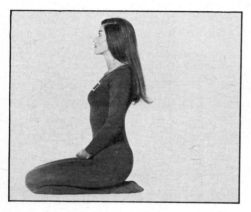

1  Sit on the heels, with the back straight and head erect.

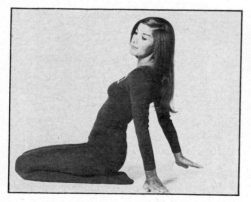

2  Carefully walk back on the hands, so that the weight is transferred gradually.

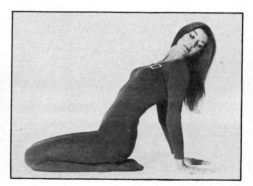

3  Place the hands about eight to ten inches away from the feet, with the fingers pointing away from you and the palms as flat on the floor as possible. Check over your shoulders to make sure that both hands are in alignment.

4 Bring the chin down onto the chest, and, once you know the movement, close your eyes.

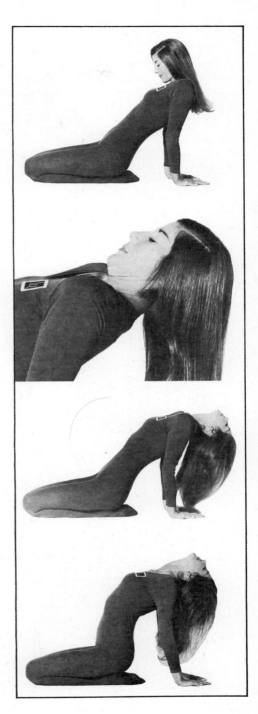

5 Slowly allow your head to go back, but keep your chin tucked in for as long as possible as this strengthens the neck muscles.

6 Allow the head to go as far back as it can without pushing it.

7 Push with the hands, and using the shoulders and the upper arms arch your spine as high as you can, but do not let the seat come off the heels. Let the head stay right back and count five keeping absolutely still.

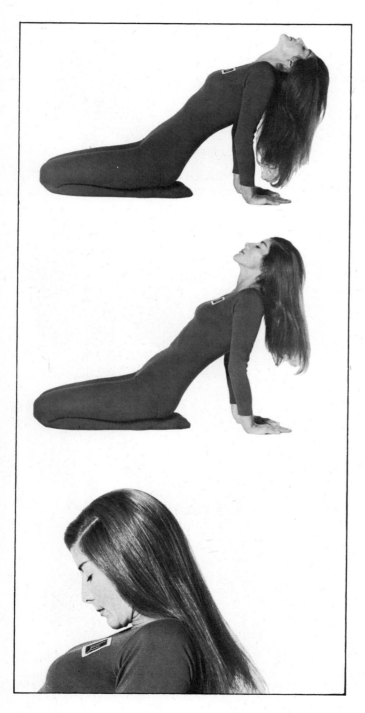

8  Slowly let the back sink down.

9  Bring the head up slowly. You may find this extremely difficult at first because the head increases in weight when blood flows into it, but in time your neck muscles will strengthen and you will be able to raise your head slowly.

10  Bring the chin back to rest on the chest, keeping the eyes closed for a few seconds.

11  Carefully transfer the weight by walking forward on the hands.

12  To relax the back completely, let the forehead come right down onto the floor in front of you and stay seated on the heels if you can.

13  Place the arms and hands in a relaxed position.

Try to stay in this relaxed position for at least a minute before repeating the movement.

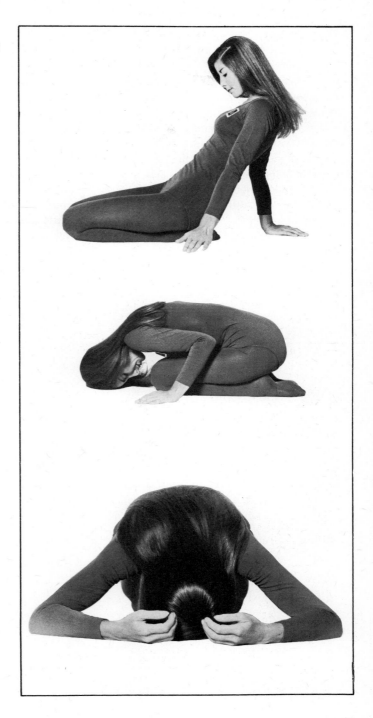

# The Cat

This movement is called the Cat because it imitates the way a cat moves, flexing the spine up and down to its extreme position.

It is a particularly valuable movement, as it works gently on the spine, to give it suppleness without putting a strain on any other part of the body. Flexing the spine this way will eliminate those aches and pains that I mentioned earlier, as well as developing greater strength and mobility throughout the back.

This movement is particularly gentle, and therefore ideal for the elderly and stiff, and for those people who have never done any back movements before. You will be helped tremendously so long as you only go as far as is comfortable in both the upward and downward positions.

As with the Backward Bend, be precise about the positioning of the hands. When you begin, make sure that your hands are placed directly underneath your shoulders as in picture 1, giving the back maximum support.

You will find that during the movement, your elbows have a tendency to bend— **don't let them**—they should remain absolutely straight all the time.

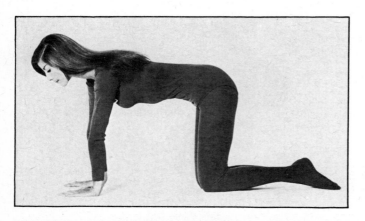

1 Come onto the hands and knees.

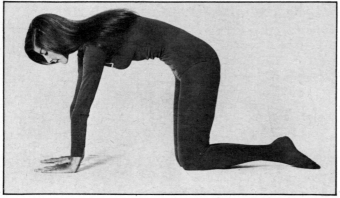

2 Slowly arch the back.

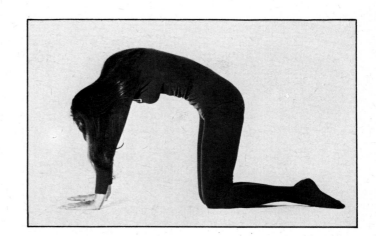

3 Arch the back a little higher. Push the pelvis gently forward and let the head relax forward.

4 Push down hard with the hands and try to get the chin onto the chest. Hold the position for a count of five, and then reverse the position.

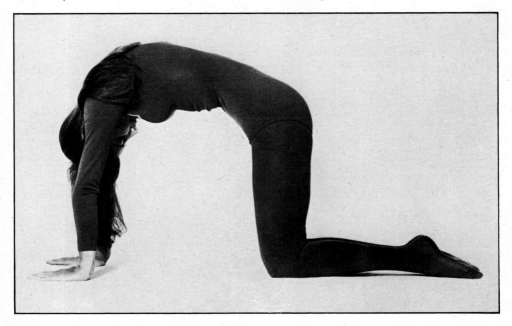

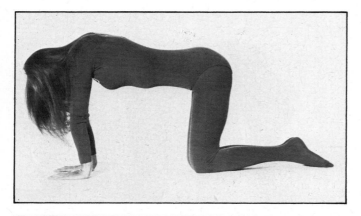

5  Let the back sink down slowly. The head stays as it is.

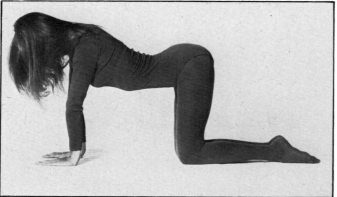

6  Push the bottom right up and out.

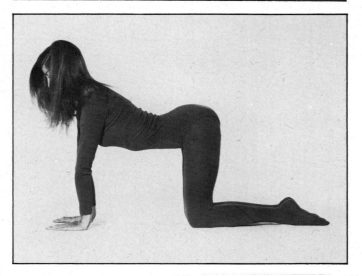

7  Start to raise the head.

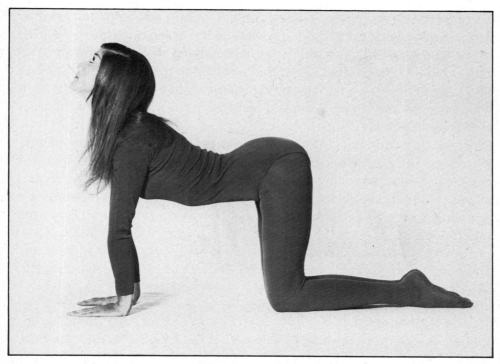

8  Raise the face and see as much of the ceiling as you can.

Hold the position for a count of five, and then repeat the entire movement once again.

Relax afterwards by sitting back on the heels, letting the forehead come down onto the floor in front of you and placing the arms and hands wherever they feel most relaxed (as shown after the Backward Bend on page 31).

Try to stay in this relaxed position for at least a minute.

# 4 Slimming and Firming

It is unfortunate that getting and keeping a slim firm body has become synonymous with physical jerks and diet sheets. Those of us that have tried this method know only too well what happens. We diet—cut down on our food—embark on whatever rigorous exercize plan we have chosen, to find that at the end of it we feel not only exhausted, but starving hungry. So it becomes a vicious circle. We exercize to burn the calories, and then eat to satisfy our increased appetites.

We are, unfortunately, a society of over-eaters, and an estimated fifty per cent of the population is overweight. This situation is one that has been exploited to the full by manufacturers of the many slimming aids and gadgets on the market, and although these seem to work miraculously for the people in the advertisements, they somehow never give you quite the same results.

The Yoga movements, on the other hand, will slim and firm the body gently and effectively, decreasing rather than increasing the appetite and stabilizing the weight once your target is reached.

## Middle-age spread
Middle-age spread is not an inevitable part of the ageing process. However, it does make you feel old when you look in the mirror and see that excess flab hanging there. You may be an extremely active person, but it is movement of the correct sort that is needed to remove that flab and then firm the body and limbs.

## Male and female problem areas
There are special movements for those areas of the body that we usually term 'problem areas'. In women it is the bottom, hips, inner and outer thighs and tummy. Men have things a little easier, because in general their problem area tends to be concentrated to just the gut. You will find these special movements on pages 42-45. Follow the instructions carefully and you will see those unwanted mounds of flesh disappearing in a matter of days.

## Hazardous to health
It is a medical fact that carrying around excess weight is bad for your health. Among other things, it puts a strain on the heart and stress on the internal organs. So lose weight the easy way by practising these movements. They are simple and pleasant to do, and will slim and firm the body the **natural** way.

# Leg Over

The Leg Over movement is marvellous for slimming and firming the tummy, waist, buttocks, hips and thighs. It entails bringing each leg over towards the opposite hand, causing an extreme twist, and stretching each side of the body from the shoulder— right down to the toes.

Execute only the modified version for now, taking care to position the arms and hands exactly as directed.

Keep the leg low when you extend it (picture 3), and do not twist or turn the head during the movement.

You will find that as you bring the right leg over, the shoulder has a tendency to raise itself up from the floor. Prevent this by pushing down hard with the palm of the right hand and keep the shoulder glued to the floor. The same applies when you do the movement with the left leg. The shoulders **must** remain on the floor in order to obtain the necessary twist and stretch in the body.

Remember that the foot does not have to touch the floor. Just take your leg over as far as it will go comfortably. The weight of your leg during the hold (for a count of five) is stretching the limbs to their maximum, and each time you perform the movement your foot will be a little closer to the floor until eventually it touches.

Once you know this movement off by heart, perform it with your eyes closed.

Relax in the Corpse for a few moments before you start the movement.

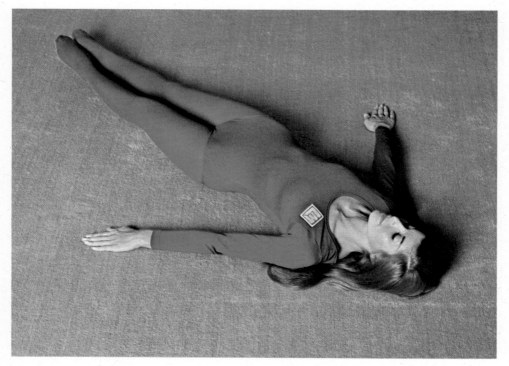

1 Bring your legs and feet together. Turn the palms of the hands towards the floor and slide the arms outwards until the hands are approximately eighteen inches from the body. Keep the elbows straight.

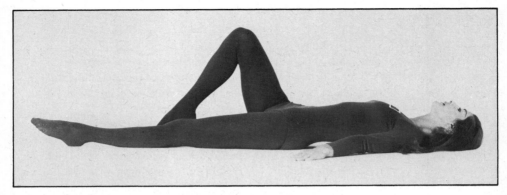

2 Slowly bend the right knee in towards the chest.

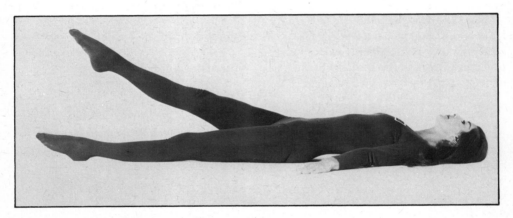

3 Extend it into the air, keeping it low.

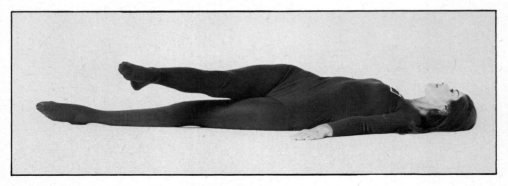

4 Bring the right foot over towards the left hand.

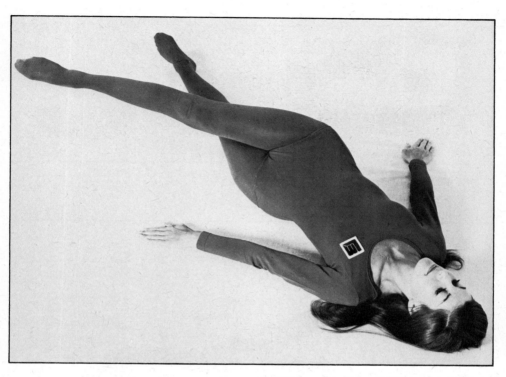

5  Hold your position still for a count of five, keeping both knees straight.

6  **Do not** let the foot crook itself inwards like this.

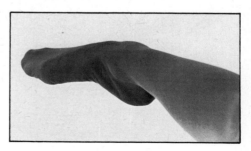

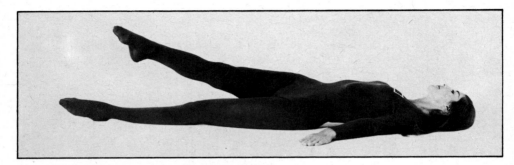

7  Take the leg slowly back over with the knee straight.

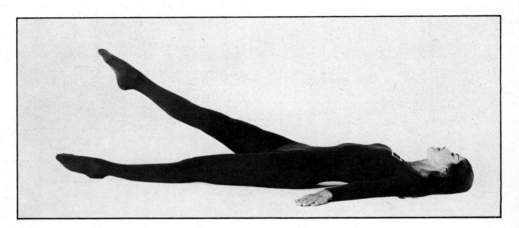

8  Until it is extended straight in front of you again.

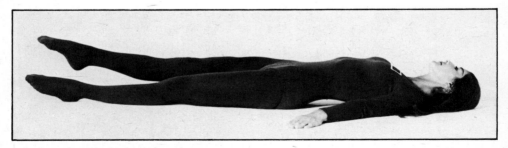

9  Lower the leg slowly to the ground.

Execute the same movement with the left leg, and then relax in the Corpse for a few seconds before performing the entire movement once again.

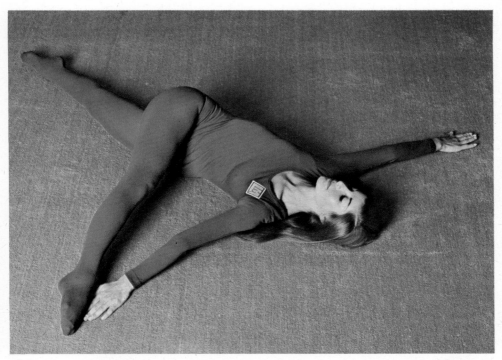

10  When you have practised for a while
and your foot touches the ground quite
comfortably in the modified position,
start to progress towards this position by
raising your arms in stages and correspond-
ingly the height of your leg. Don't rush,
and only raise your arms and legs a couple
of inches at a time.

## Male and female problem areas

These movements have been designed specifically to deal with the areas of the body where stubborn fat and flab forms. They are remarkably effective, and will show quick results. If for example you practise the appropriate movement regularly morning and evening for just one week, you will be truly amazed at the results.

# Side Raise

This is marvellously effective for the top part of the outer thigh, as well as the bottom and tummy.

Aim to raise the legs only a few inches at first (picture 2), and gradually build up to a higher raise.

Repeat the movement twice on each side.

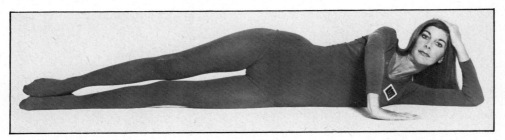

1  Lie on your side, supporting your head with your hand, and place the other hand eight to ten inches from the chest for balance.

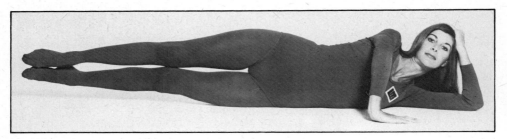

2  Raise both legs, keeping the knees straight and the feet together. Count five in this position and lower the legs slowly.

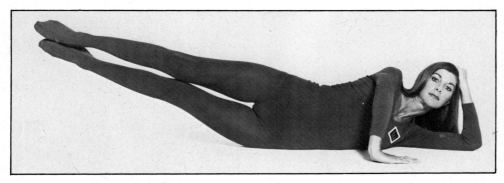

3  After a lot of practice you will be able to raise the legs to a higher position.

# Thigh Stretch

This is really a miracle movement, because it gets to those globules of fatty tissue that develop right at the top of the leg—inside the thighs—as no other movement can. This is a particularly delicate part of the body that is not used to being stretched, so be very careful with yourself and don't expect more than a very slight movement to begin with.

Don't jerk as you push your knees down. Press them down gently until you become aware of the stretch inside the thighs— hold only for a couple of seconds—and let the knees come up again.
Repeat the movement four times.

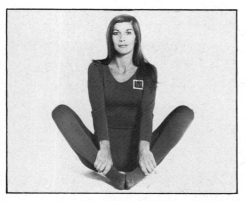

1  Sit on the floor. Bend the knees and bring the soles of the feet together.

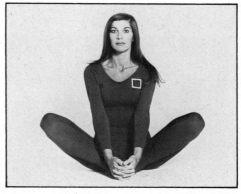

2  Interlock the fingers and place them around the toes, straightening the back as much as you can.

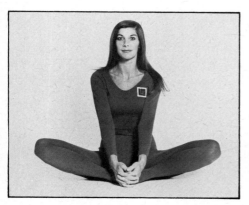

3  Gently and slowly push the knees down. Hold for only a couple of seconds and let the knees come up again.

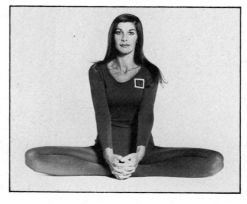

4  Gradually the knees will go further and further down, until they are flat on the floor.

# Back Push-up

Young, old, fat or thin, so many men seem to have a gut problem. In order to disperse this roll of surplus flesh, you must move it.

There are numerous exercizes and movements that work on the abdomen, but these are of no value if your aim is to rid yourself of that bulge beneath the chest. This movement really does **move** that area, and will not only eliminate surplus flesh in the gut, but also strengthen your back and shoulders.

Remember to go into the Corpse position for just a few seconds before you begin.

Raise the back slowly, holding in your comfortable position for a count of five, and then lower the back slowly. Raise four times before extending the legs, bringing the arms back to your sides and going once again into the Corpse for a few moments before you stand up.

Your shoulders **must** stay on the ground all the time.

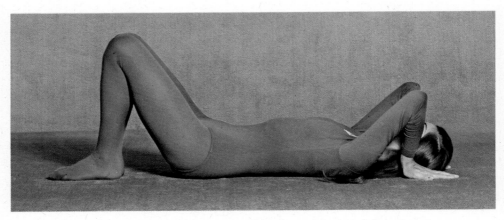

1 Bend the knees. Bring the feet in close to the body, and the hands beside the ears.

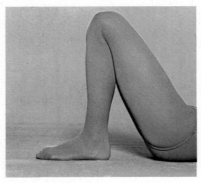

2 Keep the knees and feet together all the time.

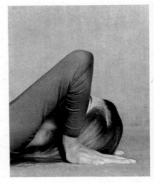

3 Try to get your palms flat on the floor, fingers pointing away from you. Make sure that your elbows are pointing straight up—not out at angles.

44

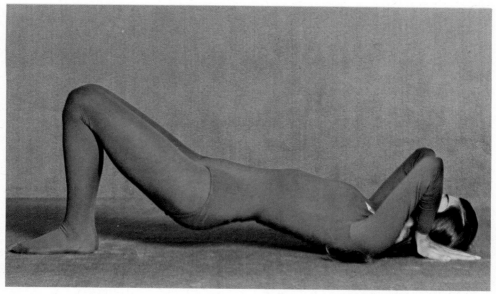

4  Push down with the hands and feet and raise the body just a few inches.

Hold for a count of five, then lower slowly.

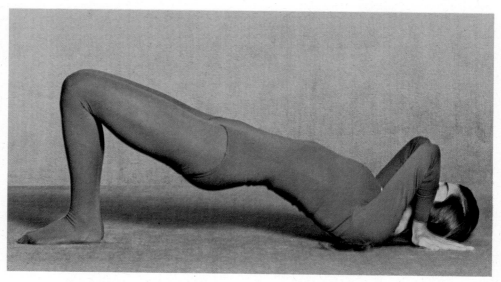

5  After some practice you can raise the body a little more, until eventually a higher raise is attained.

Increase your raise very gradually, coming up only to a height that you know you can hold still for the count of five.

# Slow Motion Firming

This is a particularly valuable movement, as it slims and firms practically every part of the body and is done in continuous slow motion. That means that there is no holding or stopping during the movement.

Once you have started the movement, execute it twice without pausing in between, and then relax at the end by going into the Corpse for a few moments.

Remember to move slowly and smoothly, keeping your knees and feet together all the time.

**Caution** Do not attempt to extend your legs as high as is shown in picture 3. Start in a much more modified position approximately eighteen inches off the floor. Also take the legs only at mid-calf and then gradually you can work down to the ankle (see picture 8).

Begin by lying down flat on your back in the Corpse posture.

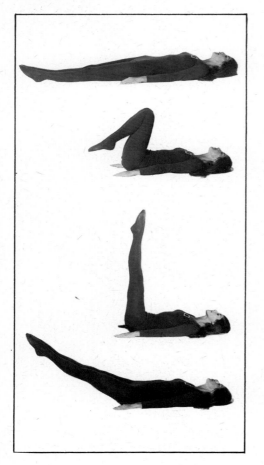

1 Bring feet together and turn palms of hands towards floor.

2 Bend knees in towards chest.

3 Extend legs into the air.

4 Lower legs slowly to the ground.

5  As soon as they touch, reach forward with arms and try to sit up without using the hands.

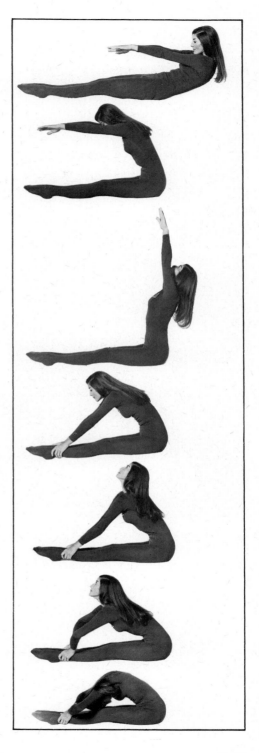

6  Until the arms are extended over the legs.

7  Raise arms above head and straighten back. Look up.

8  Bring arms down and firmly take hold of the legs (about mid-calf).

9  Raise chin as high as you can.

10  Pull on legs, letting elbows go out (bringing base of back further forward).

11  Gently let the head relax forward.

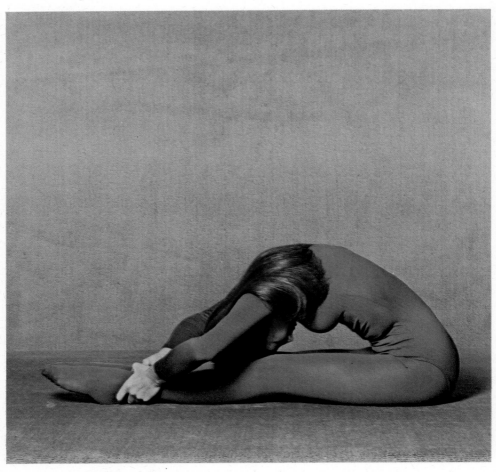

12 Now you are ready to start lying down slowly without using your hands.

13 Straighten your elbows, but keep the chin on the chest.

14 Roll slowly back down spine, hands on the thighs to keep the shoulders rounded.

15 Keep rolling back slowly—pushing down hard with the feet.

16 When your head touches the floor, put the palms of the hands onto the floor ready to repeat the entire movement once again.

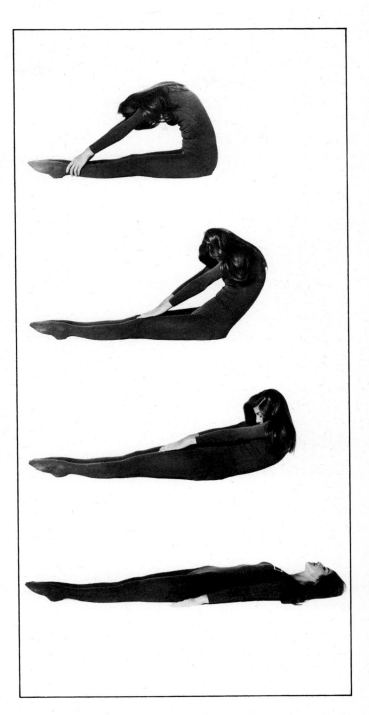

# 5 Look Better—Feel Better

We are all concerned with the way we look, and we know that looking good makes us feel good. Unfortunately, we have been brainwashed into believing that in order to look good we have to use all manner of creams, lotions and cosmetics. However, if you want to acquire and keep a good complexion, prevent or eliminate wrinkles and sagging skin, good muscle tone in the face and neck is **vital**. No amount of creams and cosmetics— however good—can work effectively. You have to get the facial muscles working from the inside by simply making them move.

Children move their faces when they talk, and they are a delight to watch because they are so uninhibited about showing their emotions on their faces. However, as we get older, we tend to become less inclined to show our feelings and our facial expressions become more and more subtle, until eventually we are moving just our lips and our eyes with perhaps the occasional smile.

I am going to show you some simple movements that not only get those facial muscles working, tightening and improving the condition of the skin, but also work on the neck, the eyes, the jaw and the tongue. There is also a movement to improve the condition of the hair, but first I would like to show you this highly valuable breathing technique that has proved to be remarkably successful in relieving conditions such as insomnia, headaches, migraine, sinusitis, asthma, nervous tension and depression.

## Alternate Nostril Breathing

This breathing technique is easily the most perfect **natural tranquilizer** that I have ever come across.

From my own personal experience in teaching, I know how effective this technique can be when used in place of sleeping tablets and other tranquilizing drugs. Students who were addicted to sleeping tablets and had suffered from insomnia for years were cured of both the addiction and the condition by using this method to get to sleep. Likewise, habitual users of tranquilizers were able to kick the tablet habit.

Let me explain how and why this technique works so well as a tranquilizer. The three vital ingredients needed for sleep, namely a relaxed body, deep even breathing, and a clear mind, are provided by breathing to a rhythm of 4-4-4-4 counts: (1) inhaling through one nostril; (2) closing both nostrils and holding the breath; (3) exhaling through the other nostril; (4) remaining without breath. You would then repeat—but inhaling through the nostril that you just breathed out of—thus forming a complete rotation. The body is forced to relax, because you are breathing so deeply and evenly, and you are concentrating so completely on counting that all other thoughts are automatically erazed from your mind, and sleep comes.

For the relief of insomnia, I suggest that you execute three rotations, sitting up in bed with the legs extended so that you can lie straight back afterwards.

Make your breathing slow, and try to measure your breath so that you take all four counts to breathe in and out. After a few rounds, you will feel the correct and comfortable speed at which to count. The eyes should be closed once you know the movement.

For the details of how to use the same technique to relieve many other conditions, refer to the Index on pages 91-95.

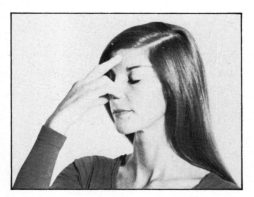

1  Place the right hand on the forehead. Use the thumb to close the right nostril and the third and fourth fingers to close the left nostril.

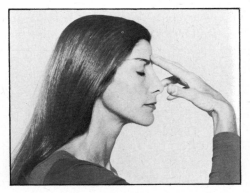

2  Breathe in through the right nostril for four counts.

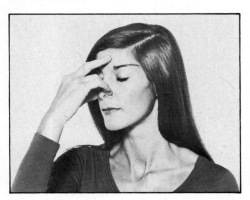

3  Close both nostrils for the next set of four.

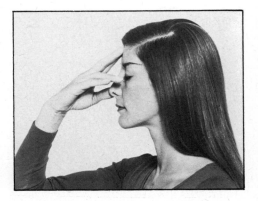

4  Exhale through the left nostril for four counts.
Release both nostrils, remaining without breath for the fourth set of four.
Repeat, breathing in through the left nostril.

# The Lion

So called because, as you will see from the pictures, it does rather resemble a lion roaring.

You may feel a little foolish at first, sitting on the floor and sticking your tongue out, but don't be put off. After you have executed the movement seriously a couple of times and felt the blood coming into your face, your eyes becoming clearer and a sensation of freshness and cleanliness in the mouth, you will not be concerned with how you look.

The benefits of this movement are many. It is extremely effective in working the facial muscles, tightening and firming the flesh.

Do not be afraid to push the tongue right out and down, and keep the jaw as wide open as you can for the count.

**Note**
**Do not** attempt the Lotus position as shown. It takes some time before this position can be attained comfortably— so just sit with the legs simply crossed.

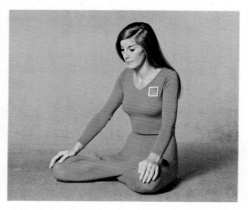

1 Sit with the legs crossed, and rest the palms of the hands on the knees.

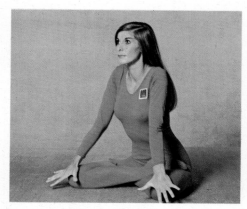

2 Push down with the hands, spreading the fingers, and widen the eyes.

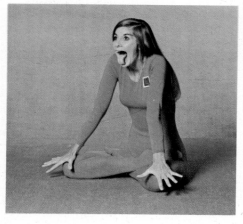

3 Push the tongue right out and down as far as you can.

Count five holding still. Then retract the tongue, relax the arms and hands and just close your eyes and rest the face for a few seconds before repeating the movement.

Execute the movement four times in all.

# Jaw Lift

This movement not only exercizes the jaw and the face, but it disperses the fleshy deposit that develops underneath the chin.

It is important to remember that this movement is divided into three parts.

First let the jaw drop open.

Then make the bottom part of the jaw really jut out.

Then take the bottom teeth right up and over the top teeth and lip.

You then let the jaw drop open again and repeat.

Keep the head back as far as it can go, without pushing it, whilst doing this movement.

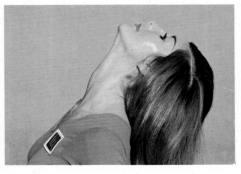

1 Let the head go back.

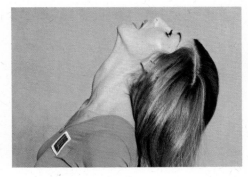

2 Let the jaw drop open.

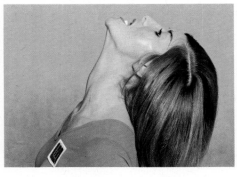

3 Make the bottom part of the jaw jut right out.

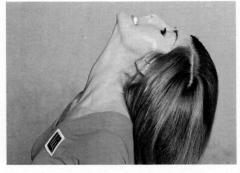

4 Take the bottom teeth right up and over the top teeth and lip. Hold only for a second or two and let the jaw drop open again.

Repeat the movement four times in all, then bring the head erect and swallow once —a really big swallow, as this movement produces a lot of saliva in the mouth.

Then bring the chin down onto the chest, close your eyes and relax the face completely for a few moments.

53

# Scalp Tugs

In order for the hair to look good and be healthy, blood must get to the hair follicles to feed them. If it doesn't, the hair dies and subsequently falls out.

Thinning and loss of hair are partially hereditary, but they can also be attributed to the fact that the scalp may be tight and the blood is not able to circulate freely. Movement of the scalp and stimulation of the blood flow is therefore very important to keep both scalp and hair in good condition. Unfortunately, the closest most people get to this is when they have a shampoo—but moving the scalp is not difficult when you know how.

This movement really does move the scalp, and if you practise regularly, you will see a marked improvement in both the appearance and the condition of your hair.

The fingers are pushed hard into the hair against the scalp, and fists are made of the hands, gripping the hair as close to the roots as possible. **The fists must be tight against the scalp**—if they are not, as you tug you will be pulling your hair. This is not only painful, but it does not enable you to move the scalp sufficiently.

Do not tug hard to begin with—just get the feeling of being able to move your scalp forward and backward slowly. As you practise, gradually increase the speed of the forward and back movements, taking care not to hurt yourself, until the movement becomes a firm tug.

Execute the movement forward and backward four times in the front of the head, then take the hands out of the hair. Repeat in the back section of the head, by placing the fingers behind the ears and pushing up towards the crown of the head.

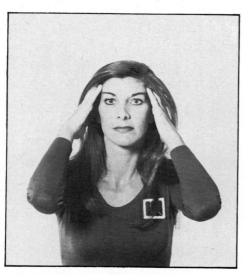

1 Place the fingers at the temples.

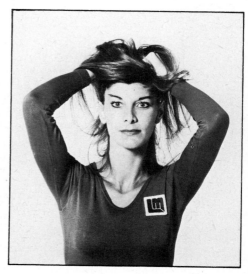

2 Push the fingers hard into the hair and make fists of the hands as close to the roots as possible.

54

3 Tug forwards.

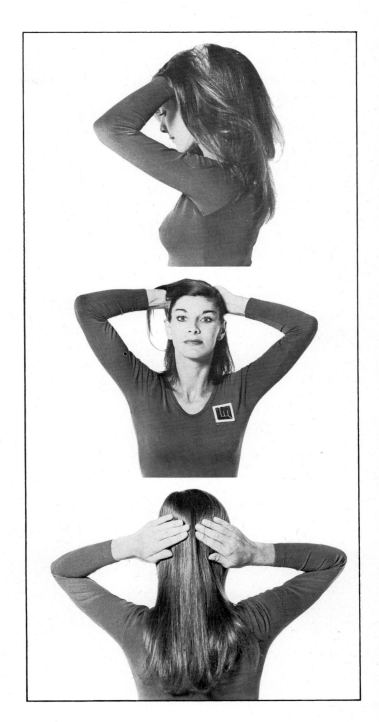

4 Tug backwards.

5 Repeat in the back
section of the head.

# 6 Legs and Feet

Most of us tend to take our legs and feet for granted, and to a certain extent we abuse them.

We are on them for much of the day and they are carrying our body weight around from one place to another. This builds up a lot of pressure in both legs and feet and can lead to all sorts of problems, the most common being aching legs and tired feet. Usually, the most we ever do for this condition is either to sit down and take the weight off our feet, or to stick them in a hot bath. What we don't seem to realize is that to refresh and relax the legs and feet properly, the pressure of blood has to be relieved. This means relaxing all the muscles and joints and allowing the blood to flow freely in and out of the legs and feet. This is achieved by simply raising the legs and inverting them.

Constant pressure of blood can also cause many vein and artery conditions, including varicose veins, so it really is worth while to set aside just a few minutes in the day to let your legs and feet **relax completely**.

## Shoulder Stand

One of the most effective ways of inverting the legs and feet and relaxing them completely is the Shoulder Stand. However, do not be put off by pictures you may have seen of people balanced vertically on their shoulders, because for the purposes of relaxing the legs and the feet you have only to execute this first modified position.

By going into this very modified position, the legs are raised sufficiently to give complete relief and relaxation to the legs and feet, but as you will see the trunk remains on the floor.

After you have been practising this for a while—should you want to—start to work towards the second modified position (page 58). Do not rush—and only go on to the next position after a lot of practice, ensuring that you have built up the strength to execute the movement with control.

Begin by lying in the Corpse position for a few moments.

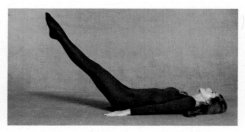

1 Bring the legs and feet together and turn the palms of the hands towards the floor. By pushing down hard with the hands, raise the legs off the floor.

2 Raise the legs with the knees straight and the feet together.

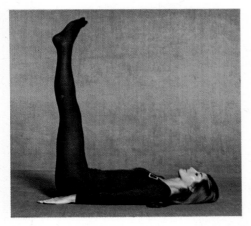

**3 First modified position.**
Relax leg and feet muscles and hold for
a count of ten—then lower slowly to
the ground.

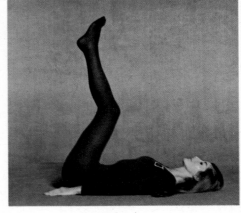

4 If you find it difficult to keep your knees
straight for the count of ten, then let them
bend a little.

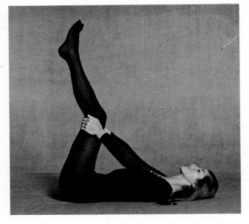

5 If you feel you want to support the legs
with the hands—that's fine.

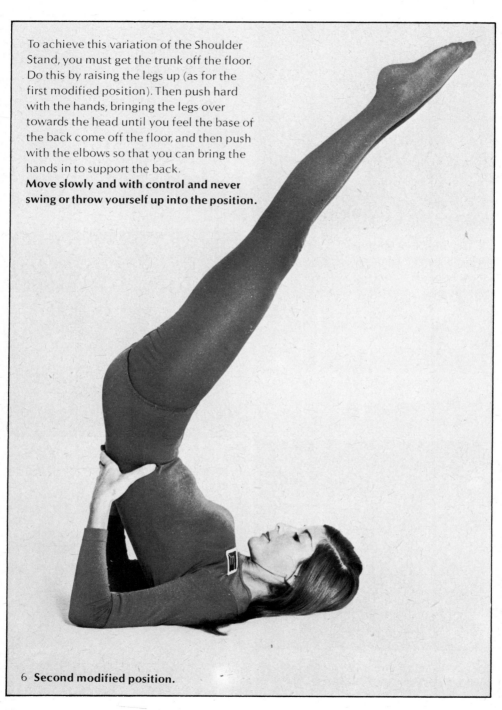

To achieve this variation of the Shoulder Stand, you must get the trunk off the floor. Do this by raising the legs up (as for the first modified position). Then push hard with the hands, bringing the legs over towards the head until you feel the base of the back come off the floor, and then push with the elbows so that you can bring the hands in to support the back.
**Move slowly and with control and never swing or throw yourself up into the position.**

6 **Second modified position.**

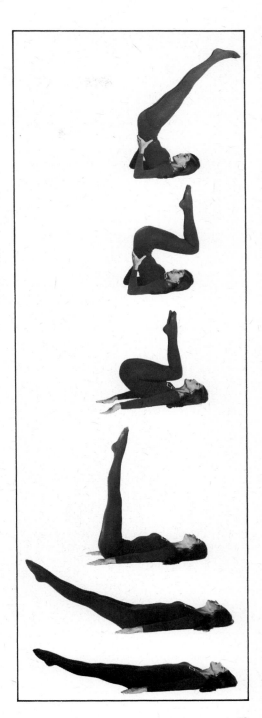

7 Gently relax the leg and feet muscles, and hold the position still for a count of ten, breathing slowly and deeply.

8 Tense the leg and feet muscles and slowly bend the knees in towards the chest, tucking the feet in as much as you can.

9 Put the hands back onto the floor, and start to roll **slowly** back down the spine.

10 Extend the legs, keeping the head on the floor.

11 Lower the legs slowly to the ground, knees straight, feet together, and when they touch, relax in the Corpse position for a few moments.

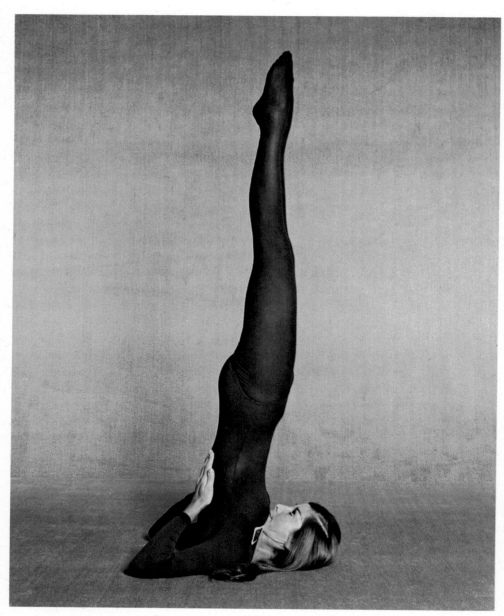

12  The Completed Shoulder Stand with the body and legs going straight up in a vertical line.

13  After many years of practice, it may be possible to build up sufficient strength, so that the hands can be taken away and the back is supporting the body unaided.

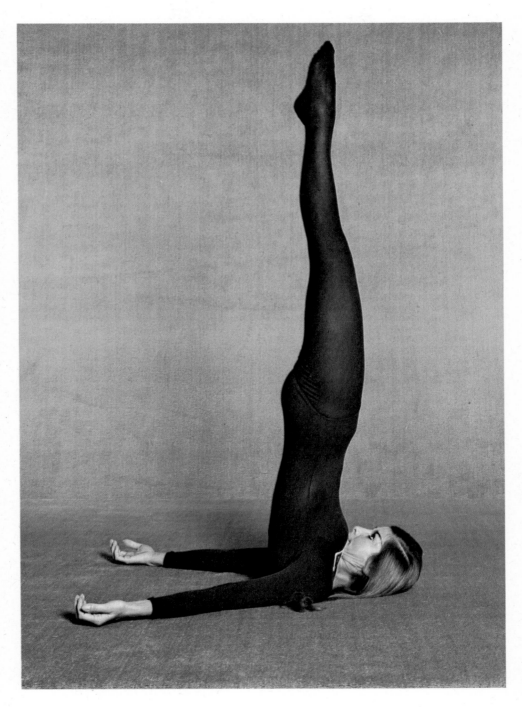

# Leg Pulls

This movement enables you to work separately on each leg, reducing any surplus flesh and firming the legs and thighs. It also gently stretches one of the tightest muscle areas of the body—the hamstring muscles at the backs of the legs.

To begin with, take hold of the leg on or just below the knee. Gradually as you practise, you can go further and further down the leg, until eventually you are able to take hold of the ankle, as shown in picture 4.

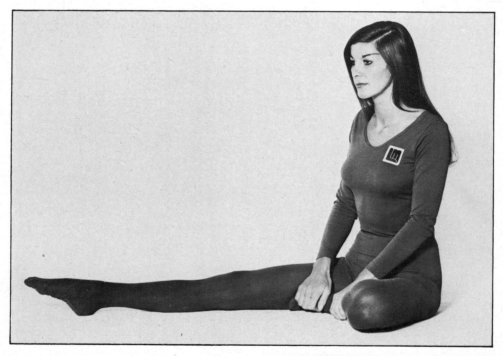

1 Sit on the floor with the right leg extended and bring the left foot in as close to the body as you can. (The sole of the left foot goes along the inside of the right thigh.)

Your knee will probably be off the floor like this at first, which is fine. Don't try to push it down. As you practise you will find that it goes further and further until eventually it touches the floor.

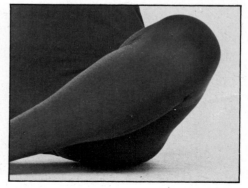

2 Extend the arms over the leg.

3 Bring them straight up above the head.

4 Bring the arms down and take a firm grip on the leg with both hands (on or just below the knee).

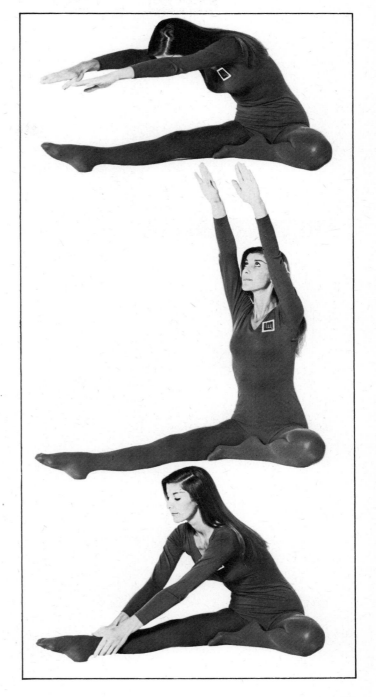

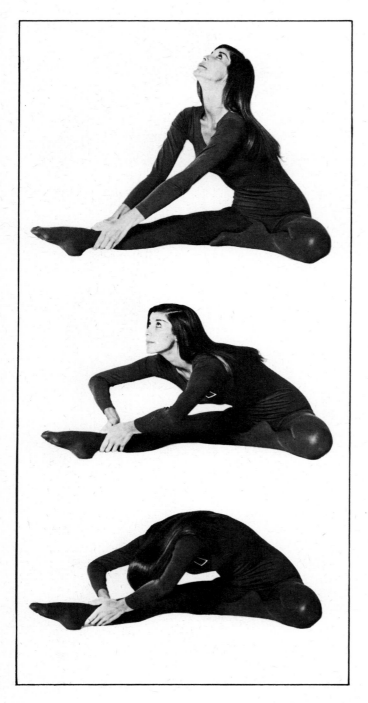

5  Raise the chin as high as you can.

6  Pull on the leg, letting the elbows go out until you become aware of the stretch at the back of the leg.

7  Gently let the head relax forward.

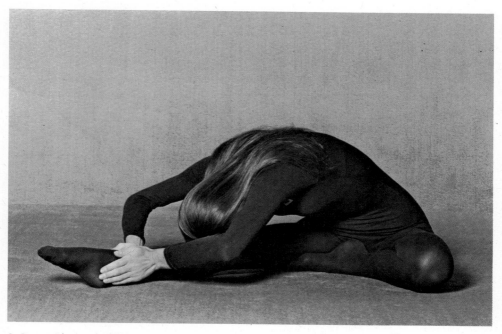

8  Remember to hold absolutely still for the count of five in the finished position. Allow the head to relax completely over and make sure that your elbows **go out — not down**.

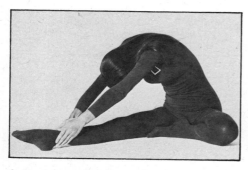

9  Straighten the elbows, but let the head stay relaxed forward.

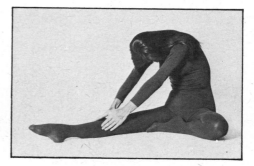

10  Slide the hands up the leg, straighten the back and raise the head, ready to repeat the entire movement again.

Execute the movement twice on each leg.

# Foot Rotations

The muscles, ligaments and joints in our toes, feet and ankles are sadly neglected. It seems that only when we have pulled a muscle or ligament, twisted an ankle or dislocated a joint, do we become aware of how important our feet are.

Few people have the time or the desire to do much walking today, and many of those that do are causing more harm than good by inhibiting the natural movement of the foot in the confines of modern-day footwear. So to combat this and keep the muscles and joints in the toes, feet and ankles working correctly, this foot rotation movement is simple but extremely effective.

Rotate the foot slowly ten times, taking care to keep the leg absolutely still and the knee straight. You will find this a little difficult at first as your leg will probably move as you rotate the foot. Don't let it. Also, make sure that you take your foot to its extreme in each of the four positions, and try not to cut corners.

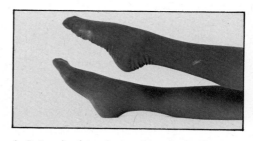

2  Point the foot down towards the floor.

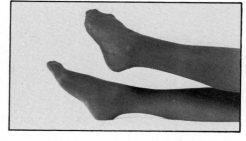

3  Crook the foot in as far as it will go.

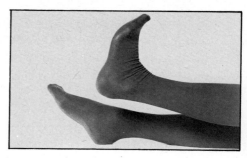

4  Right up so that the heel is pushed forward and the toes are back.

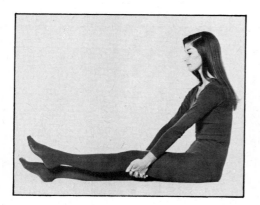

1  Sit on the floor with both legs extended in front of you. Raise one leg just a few inches, and support it by interlocking the fingers underneath it.

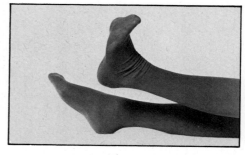

5  Right over to the other side and then down towards the floor again, ready to repeat.

After repeating ten rotations, repeat with the other foot.

# 7 Life with Yoga

So far I have shown you how to use the different Yoga movements to tackle and help relieve many of today's common ailments and problems, and you will find them most effective in doing just that. However, the Yoga movements are extremely versatile, and although I have recommended specific movements for specific maladies and conditions, those very same movements can be used beneficially in many other ways.

The Tension Release in Chapter 2, for example, shown for relieving tension at the top of the spine, is also a marvellous movement to do for developing the chest and firming the bust. Likewise, the last movement in Chapter 6, Foot Rotations, is not only good for working out the stiffness of the joints in the toes and feet, but it is also very effective for slimming the legs and ankles. In the same way, the postures and movements shown in the following pages can be used in many different ways. For details of the many benefits that each movement will bring, see the index on pages 91-95.

Practise and enjoy the Yoga movements, not only for specific conditions, but to improve and so get more enjoyment out of your everyday life.

Bear in mind also that the movements need be practised for no other reason than the fact that you get pleasure out of doing them.

The more you practise, the more you will come to appreciate that Yoga reigns supreme in providing the most perfect and natural form of body movement as well as mental and physical relaxation.

Your life with Yoga can be nothing but richer, used whenever and however you like, and it will make you aware that your body is not just a part of you —**it is you.**

# Standing Stretch

This movement is invaluable whenever you feel you need a really good stretch, whether it is first thing in the morning or at any time during the day. It stretches the body and limbs by bending forward and back and then side to side, but only going to your comfortable maximum in each of the four positions—**which means not straining.**

The actual movement begins over the page, but before you start, study and familiarize yourself with these four preparatory positions, and practise them. When you know them by heart you will be able to turn the page and come into the correct starting position (picture 5) so that you can then execute the entire movement without stopping.

Remember to move slowly and smoothly, and always come back to the upright position before bending in another direction. Try to keep the upper arms level with the ears as shown, and keep the elbows and knees straight.

When you start, go only to the first position shown in each direction. As you practise, you will be able to go further and further as your body stretches.

After executing the movement, relax the body forward letting the head, arms and hands just hang for a few seconds. Then straighten up slowly and, if you wish, repeat the entire movement once again.

**Note** Although it may appear from the pictures that I turn round after the forward and back movements, this is just to show the position of the body more clearly. You should not alter your position all the way through.

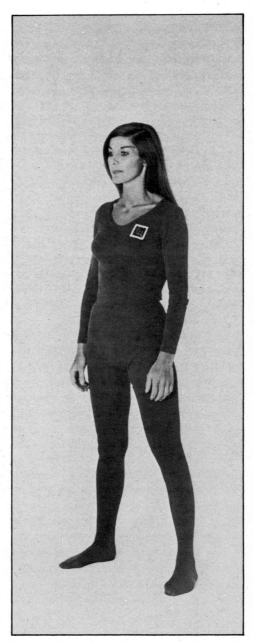

1 Stand with the feet approximately twenty inches apart, arms at your sides and the head erect.

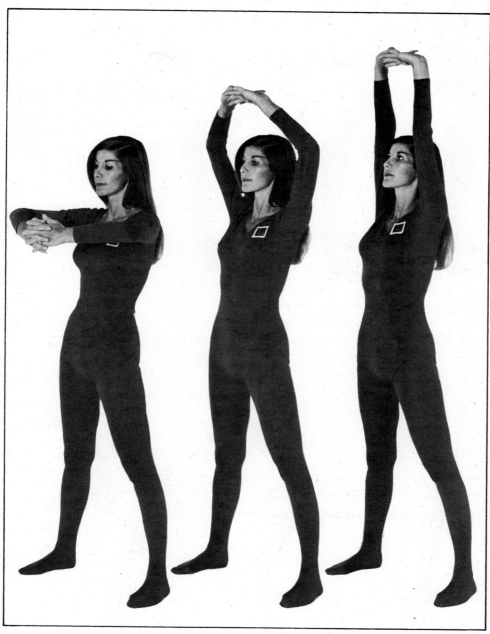

2 Interlock the fingers.

3 Turn the palms of the hands away from you and up towards the ceiling.

4 Gently straighten the elbows.

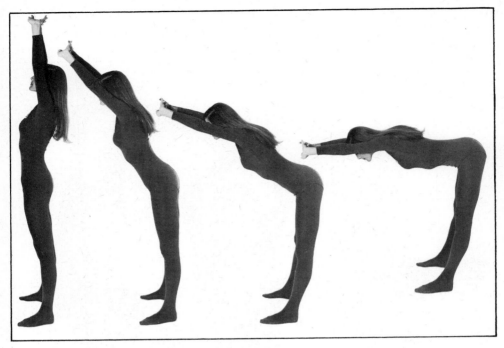

5  Upright starting
position.

6  Bend forward just a little from the hips,
and straighten up slowly.

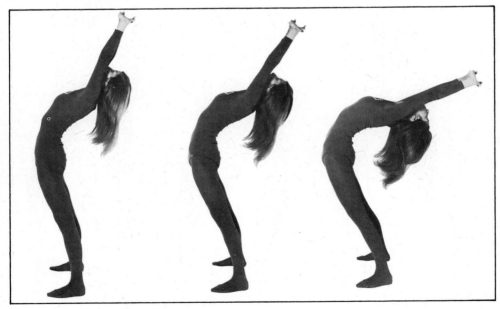

7  Go back from the hips, just a little way,
and raise your eyes so that you can see
the ceiling. Straighten up slowly.

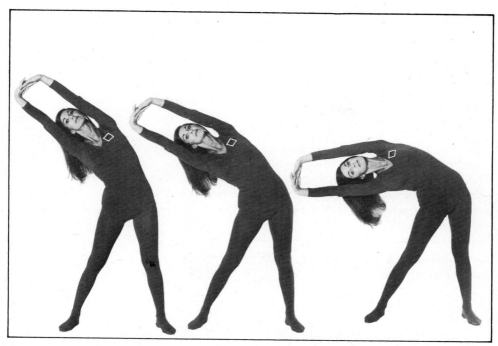

8 Go gently over to your right, and
straighten up slowly.

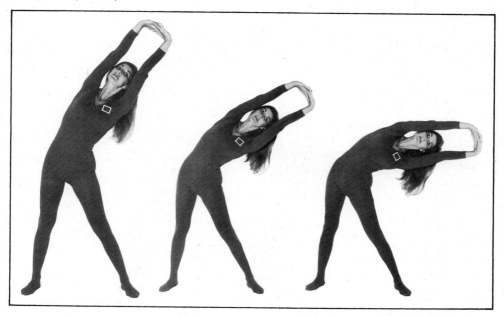

9 Over to your left, straighten up slowly
and then relax the body forward.

# The Cobra

This is a marvellous movement for the spine, arching it gently from the very top right down to the base of the back.

It is not a push-up—the hips and abdomen remain on the floor. Your objective should be to arch the back as much as you can rather than to straighten the elbows, although in time the elbows will straighten.

Execute the movement twice, moving extremely slowly.

1 Lie on the stomach and relax completely before you begin by turning the face so that the cheek rests on the floor. Let the heels fall open and let the elbows bend, relaxing the fingers and the shoulders.

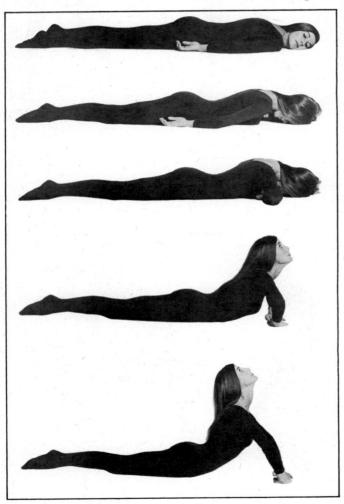

2 Bring the feet together and rest the forehead on the floor, bringing it right up onto the hairline if you can.

3 Bring the hands in underneath the shoulders, palms towards the floor, and try to get the elbows on the floor.

4 Slowly raise the face to see the ceiling.

5 By pushing down hard with the hands, start to arch the back slowly. Stop when you reach your comfortable limit and hold for five.

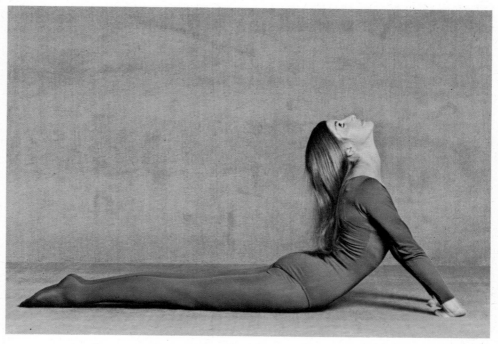

6  In time your elbows will straighten completely.

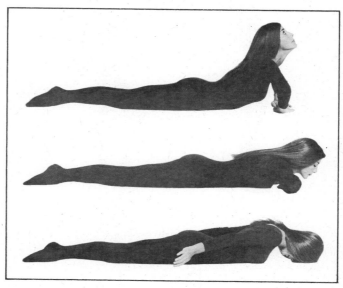

7  Let the back come down by slowly bending the elbows, but keep the head back.

8  When the elbows touch the floor bring the head slowly down.

9  Place the forehead on the floor again and bring the arms back to your sides.

Then go into the position of relaxation for a few moments (picture 1) before repeating the entire movement once again.

# Balance Posture

Most people find it extremely difficult to balance, and even more difficult to concentrate properly. By practising this simple movement you can achieve both of these vital things. I say vital because a sense of balance is essential for improving and maintaining good posture whether you are walking, sitting or standing, and the ability to concentrate completely at will is a phenomenon that eludes most people.

By practising this seemingly insignificant movement, you will find that you are forced to use **all** of your concentration, for the instant your mind starts to wander you will lose balance. The result is that your mind becomes trained to shut out any surrounding distractions, and this will become invaluable in your everyday life both at work and leisure.

If you lose your balance, come out of the position and relax for a few seconds, then start slowly again from the beginning.

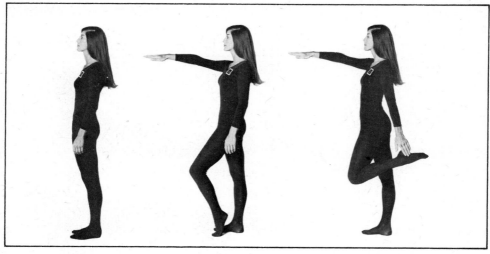

1  Stand with the legs and feet together, back straight, head erect.

2  Raise the right arm slowly to shoulder level and flex the left knee, putting the weight onto the right leg.

3  When you feel you have the balance, gently raise the left foot and try to take hold of it with the left hand.

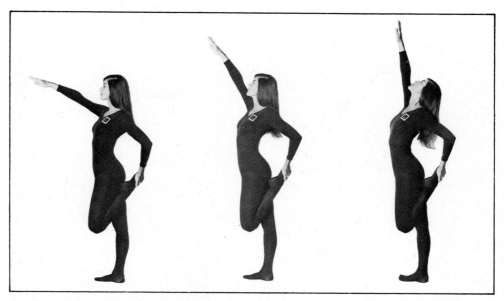

4 Raise the right arm a few inches, and by bending the left elbow draw the foot in a little closer to the body.

5 As you practise, you will find you can raise the arm higher and higher.

6 In time you can bring your arm straight above your head.

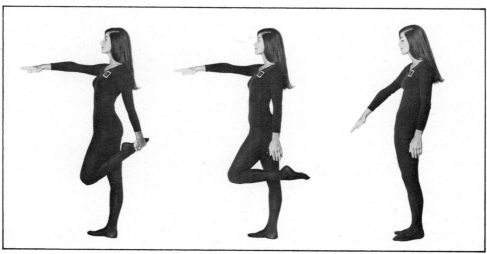

7 Hold the position for only a few seconds, then allow the left elbow to straighten slowly and bring the right arm back down to shoulder level.

8 Try to release the left foot gently and with control so that it doesn't spring out of the hand and cause you to lose balance, and bring it slowly down to the floor.

9 Bring the right arm slowly back down to your side.
   Repeat movement on the other side.

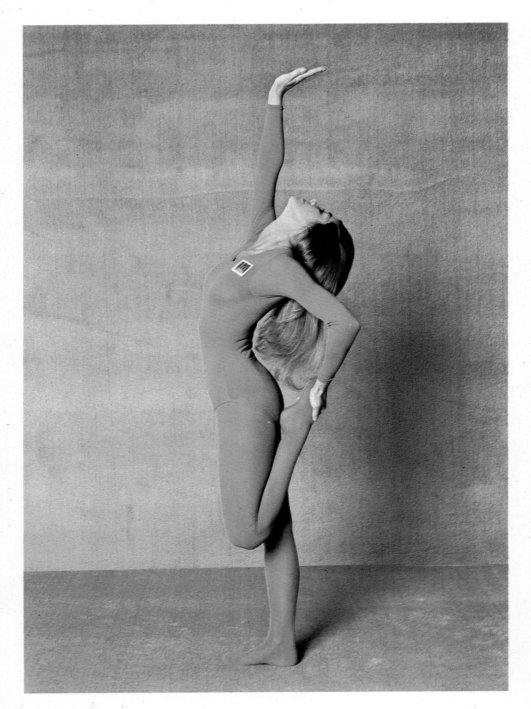

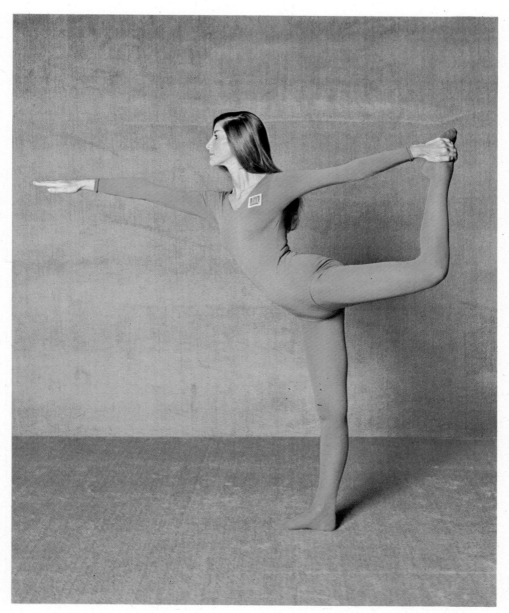

10 Eventually you will be able to come into this extreme upright position with the head back.

11 This very advanced variation is achieved by extending the arm and the leg as far as possible, while still keeping hold of the foot.

# Scissors

I have called this movement the scissors, because, as you will see, the arms open and close at corresponding speeds, exactly as do the blades of a pair of scissors.

Begin by standing straight, back up and head erect. Place the feet about five or six inches apart, but don't let the toes point outwards as this may affect your balance.

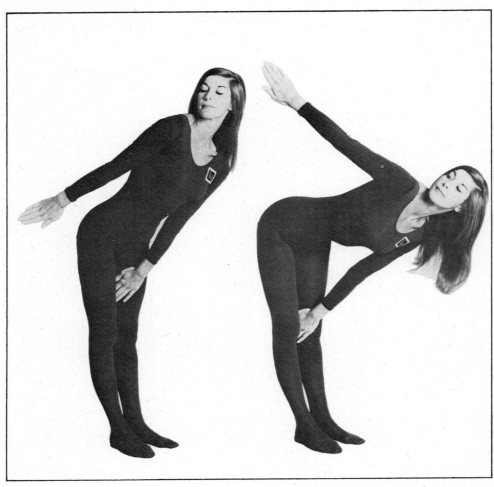

1  Slide the palm of the left hand down the inside of the left leg, raising the right arm slowly at the same time.
Keep both elbows straight and the eyes on the back of the raised hand.

2  Stop in this position with the left hand just below the knee and the right arm and hand at the corresponding height.
Hold the position absolutely still for a count of five.

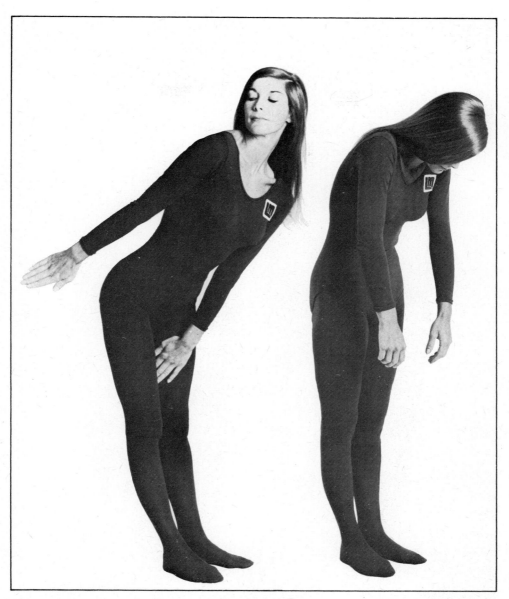

3 Slowly begin to slide the left hand back
up the leg, and lower the right arm and
hand so that both arms are moving at
exactly the same pace.

4 When both hands reach the tops of the
thighs, relax the head and shoulders over
for a few moments before repeating the
same movement on the other side.
Then repeat once more on each side.

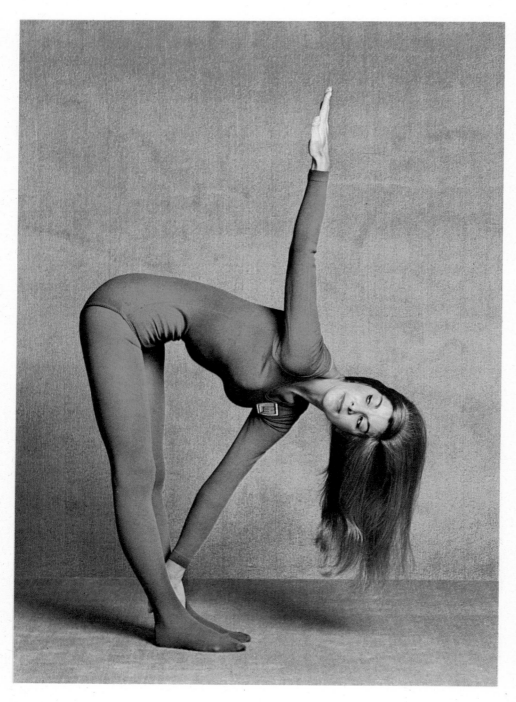

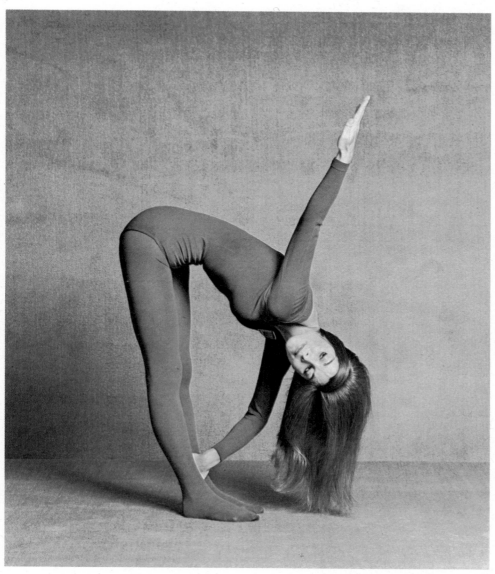

5  You will find that each time you perform
the movement the hand will go a little
further down the leg, until eventually it
will go right down comfortably to the foot
area, and the raised arm will be at a
corresponding height.

6  A more advanced variation is achieved
by pulling on the back of the leg, and
letting the elbow bend to bring the body
further over from the hips.

# The Twist

This movement is a good back strengthener and it enables you to twist the back in a rather unusual way using your own body as leverage.

It works out stiffness from the centre of the back as well as from the neck and shoulders.

As you can see it can be performed very efficiently sitting on a chair or stool, as well as on the floor, so it makes it an ideal movement to do while at work.

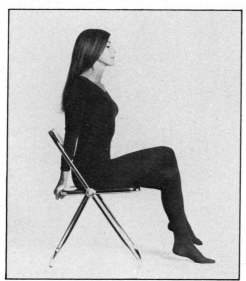

1  Sit with the legs together and the back straight.

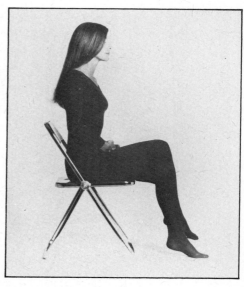

2  Cross right leg over left.

3  Grip chair behind you with right hand.

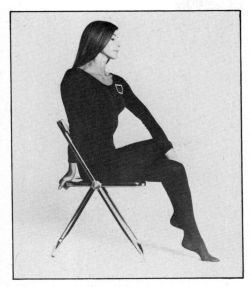

4 Bring left arm over right knee and get a firm hold of left knee, keep elbow straight if you can.

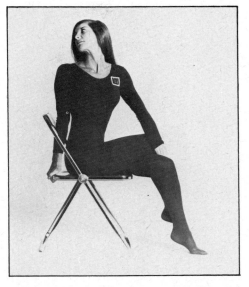

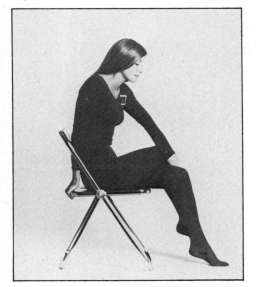

5 Now you have formed a lock with the arms and legs.
Pull hard with both hands and twist against this lock by turning the head and shoulders slowly round to the right. Try to look directly behind you, and hold the position still for a count of five.

6 Let the head and shoulders come slowly round to the front, but keep the arms and legs in position so that you can repeat the twisting movement once again.
Then uncross the legs and repeat the movement twice on the other side.

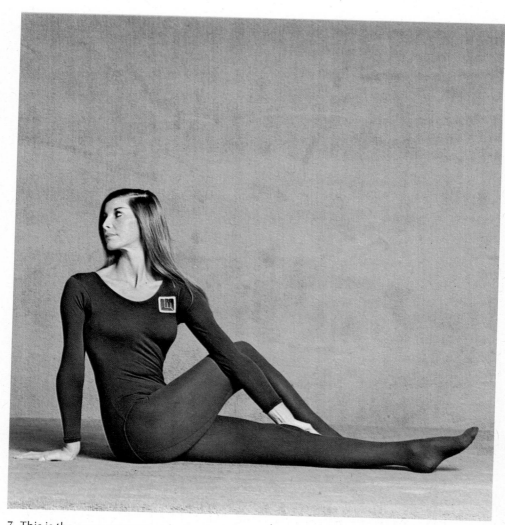

7 This is the same movement, but seated
on the floor.
Start with the legs extended out in front of
you, and follow the same instructions as for
the Twist seated on the chair. The only
difference is that you will place the right
hand on the floor behind you as shown.

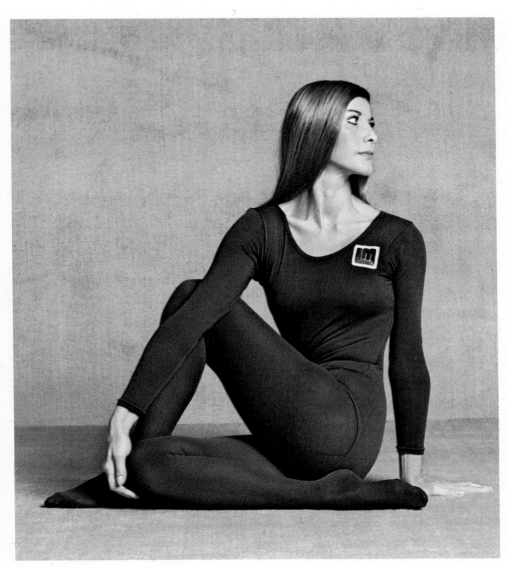

8  This position is the Full Twist, achieved
only after a lot of practice. For our purposes
the Simple Twist is sufficient, but this is
what it is ultimately leading up to.

# Elbow Snaps

Although the name of this movement may sound painful, it is not. When executed carefully and correctly it is very effective in working out the stiffness from the elbow joints and keeping them healthy.

Take the utmost care to ensure that you position your fists exactly as shown, because correct positioning is imperative if you are to receive maximum benefit from this movement.

Execute the movement slowly at first, until you are sure that your fists correspond with the positions shown. Gradually, you can use a little more impetus, until eventually you can contract the elbows sharply in as you extend the arms.

Perform this movement six times, just pausing for a second in the extended position before bending the elbows and bringing the fists in level with the chest again.

Whether you are sitting on a chair or the floor, try to sit with the back as straight as possible.

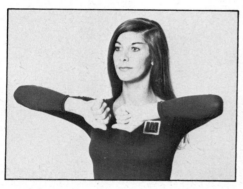

1  Make fists out of the hands and bending the elbows bring the fists in level with the chest.

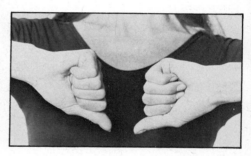

2  Make sure that the thumbs are pointing towards the floor.

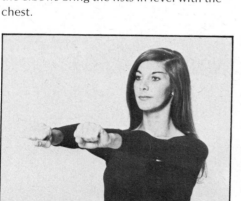

3  Extend the arms, sharply contracting the elbows in.

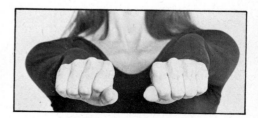

4  Make sure that the fists end square on like this.

# Finger Pulls

This movement is deceiving, because although it looks as if it is just the fingers that are being worked on, in fact it is the shoulders, back, chest, upper arms, forearms **and** the finger joints. You will be able to feel this as you execute the movement **slowly and smoothly.**

As with the Elbow Snaps, you can perform this either sitting on a chair or the floor, but make sure that the back is straight and the head erect.

Start with the elbows level with the chest and don't let them drop as you pull down with the fingers.

Keep the hands close to the body as you pull down and keep the shoulders back and down.

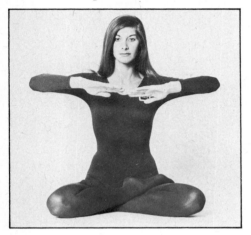

1 Bend the elbows and bring the hands in level with the chest.

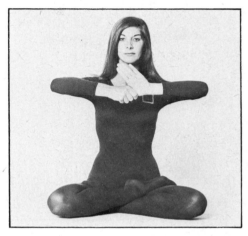

2 Turn the palm of the left hand away from you and grip the thumb firmly with the right hand.

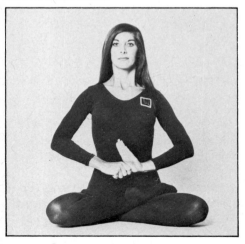

3 Pull hands in towards you and down **slowly and firmly,** pushing the chest out slightly, and don't release the thumb until the hands reach the level of the navel.

Repeat the movement with the other fingers of the left hand and then change hands, pulling the fingers of the right hand down.

**Do not** attempt the Lotus position.

# The Triangle

So called, because the body makes triangular shapes when in position.

This stretches and elongates the sides of the body, firming the torso as well as the legs and arms.

It also gives you an incredible feeling of reaching right up and over and extending the body as much as you can without causing any strain.

As with all the other postures, you are establishing stretch simply by holding still for the count in your comfortable position, so that each time you perform the movement you will find you can go a little further.

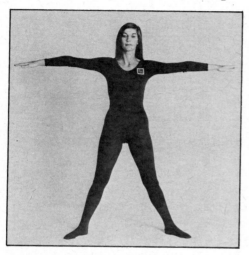

1 Stand with the feet approximately twenty inches apart and raise the arms to shoulder level.

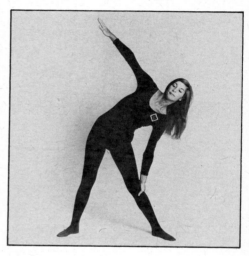

2 Keeping the elbows straight, slowly bend over to the left and grip the left leg on or just below the knee.

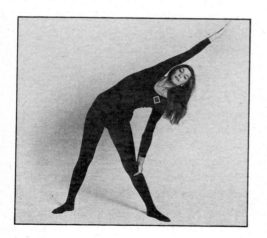

3 Bring the right arm over as close to the ear as possible and turn the palm of the right hand towards the floor.

Hold the position absolutely still for the count of five. Then straighten up and repeat on the other side.

Let the arms come down to your sides and relax for a few moments before performing the entire movement once again on both sides.

4 Eventually you will be able to come over so that the top arm is parallel with the floor.

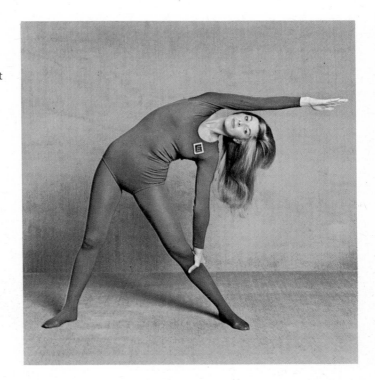

5 A more advanced variation is to bend the supporting elbow so that the body is brought over still further from the hips.

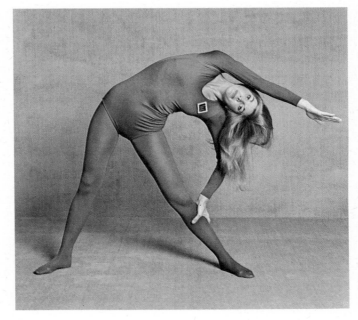

# Index of Postures and Breathing Instructions

**37-41 Leg Over**

To slim and firm the tummy, waist,
buttocks, hips and thighs.
To strengthen the shoulders and
back.
BREATHING—Breathe normally and
slowly through the nose.

**42 Side Raise**

To slim and firm the top part of the
outer thigh.
To firm the tummy and the bottom,
eliminating any surplus flesh.
To strengthen the back and the legs.
BREATHING—When in position,
take a deep breath before raising
the legs. Hold it for the count and
then exhale as you lower the legs.
(Breathe normally while relaxing
before repeating the movement.)

**43 Thigh Stretch**

To eliminate the surplus flesh right
at the top of the leg—inside the
thighs.
To stretch the knees and firm
the thighs.
BREATHING—Breathe normally and
slowly through the nose.

**44-45 Back Push-up**

To eliminate surplus flesh in the gut.
To firm and strengthen the legs,
thighs and lower back.
To strengthen the arms and
shoulders.
BREATHING—When in position,
take a deep breath before raising
the back. Hold it for the count and
exhale slowly as you lower the back.
(Breathe normally while relaxing
before repeating the movement.)

**46-49 Slow Motion Firming**

To slim and firm the arms, waist,
abdomen, bottom and legs.
To strengthen the shoulders, back
and neck.
BREATHING—Breathe normally and
slowly through the nose.

**50-51 Alternate Nostril Breathing**

To help relieve the following
conditions:
Insomnia 3
Headache 3
Migraine 5
Sinusitis 4
Asthma 4
Nasal congestion 4
Depression 3
Nervous tension 3
It will also help greatly to improve
your breathing generally, and can be
used purely as an effective relaxant.
When used for any of the above conditions,
with the exception of insomnia (see page 50),
sit either on a chair or on the floor with the
legs crossed, making sure that the back is
straight. Try to find somewhere that is both
private and quiet so that you can
concentrate completely.
Alongside each of the above conditions
there is a number, indicating how many
rotations I suggest you do to begin with.
In time, however, should you feel that you
want to do more, gradually increase by only
one rotation at a time.
Once you know the movement—**always
execute it with the eyes closed.**

BREATHING—Counting to yourself,
breathe to a rhythm of 4-4-4-4 as
instructed with the movement on
page 50.

## 52 The Lion

To work the facial muscles, firming
and tightening the flesh.
To improve the condition of the
skin and eyes.
To exercize the tongue and the jaw.
To stretch and strengthen the arms
and fingers.
BREATHING—*Breathe normally
through the nose.*

## 53 Jaw Lift

To disperse the fleshy deposit that
can develop underneath the chin,
and ensure against developing excess
flab or a double chin.
To exercize the jaw really effectively.
To stretch and strengthen the neck.
BREATHING—*Breathe normally
through the nose.*

## 54-55 Scalp Tugs

To promote healthy, shining hair.
To prevent unnecessary loss of hair.
To loosen the scalp and stimulate the
blood flow so that it can get to the
hair follicles, which is necessary to
maintain the hair and scalp in good
condition.
BREATHING—*Breathe normally
through the nose.*

## 56-61 Shoulder Stand

To relax completely the legs and feet.
To relieve pressure of blood in the
the legs.
To help ward off vein and artery
conditions, and relieve existing
conditions (subject to your doctor's
approval).
When the trunk is raised in the more
advanced versions of this position,
you will strengthen the back, the
abdomen and the legs.

To improve blood circulation in all
areas of the body and refresh and
stimulate organs and glands.
BREATHING—*Take a deep breath in
through the nose before you push
down with the hands to raise the
legs. Once in position try to breathe
deeply and as slowly as you can for
the count. Breathe normally when
coming out of the position.*

## 62-65 Leg Pulls

To stretch gently the hamstring
muscles at the backs of the legs.
To reduce any surplus flesh on the
legs or thighs.
To stretch the base of the back, and
strengthen it.
To stretch the neck, and relax and
refresh the head.
BREATHING—*When in position, as
you bring the arms up take a deep
breath in through the nose. Hold the
breath as you bring the arms down
to take the leg, raise the chin, and
pull—letting the elbows go out—
exhaling as you let the head
relax over.
(Try to remain without breath for the
hold if you can.)
Start to inhale as you slide the hands
back up the leg, and exhale as you
straighten the back before performing
the movement again.*

## 66 Foot Rotations

To work out any stiffness in the toes,
feet and ankles.
To maintain the muscles and joints
in good working order.
To slim the ankles.
To strengthen and firm the calf muscles.
BREATHING—*Breathe normally and
slowly through the nose.*

**68-71  Standing Stretch**

To stretch gently the legs, back, arms
and sides of the body, and then
relax them.
*BREATHING—When you are in
position, breathe in through the nose.
Exhale slowly as you come forward—
inhale as you come up—exhale as
you go back—inhale as you come up.
Breathe the same way for the side
bends, breathing in on the up
movement and out on the down
movement.
As you relax the body over at the
end, exhale slowly and then just
breathe normally.*

**72-73  The Cobra**

To gain strength and elasticity by
manipulating each vertebra one by
one from the very top right down to
the base of the spine.
To strengthen and firm shoulders
and arms, and to stretch the neck.
*BREATHING—Breathe normally and
slowly through the nose.*

**74-77  Balance Posture**

To improve greatly balance and
concentration.
To improve posture and gain poise.
To improve muscle control throughout entire body.
*BREATHING—Breathe normally and
slowly through the nose.*

**78-81  Scissors**

To impart a sense of balance and
co-ordination.
To stretch the backs of the legs and
the lower back.
To slim and firm the thighs and
buttocks.

*BREATHING—Take a deep breath in
through the nose, and exhale slowly
as you slide the hand down the leg.
Take another breath when in position
for the hold, but take it smoothly
and gently. From then on breathe
normally.
(Eventually you will be able to
maintain the holding position
without breath.)*

**82-85  The Twist**

To work out stiffness from the centre
of the back, neck and shoulders.
To trim the waist.
To slim and firm the arms.
*BREATHING—Breathe normally and
slowly through the nose.*

**86  Elbow Snaps**

To work out stiffness in the elbow joints.
To strengthen and firm the arms.
*BREATHING—Breathe normally
through the nose.*

**87  Finger Pulls**

To eliminate stiffness and maintain
the finger joints in good working
order.
To strengthen the back, shoulders,
upper arms, forearms and wrists.
To develop the chest and firm the bust.
*BREATHING—Breathe in as you grip
the finger—retain the breath while
you are pulling down slowly and
firmly—exhale when the hands
reach the level of the navel.*

## The Triangle

To stretch and elongate the sides of the torso.
To stretch and strengthen the legs.
To strengthen the back, shoulders and arms.

BREATHING—*As you raise the arms to start take a deep breath in through the nose, and exhale slowly as you go over to the side.*
*Take another breath in the holding position gently and smoothly, and continue the movement breathing normally.*
*Eventually you will be able to retain the holding position without breath — breathing in again as you straighten up, and exhaling as the arms become parallel with the shoulders in readiness to inhale and repeat movement on other side.*

When you have practiced and mastered the following movements, you may like to incorporate the more advanced breathing instructions as follows :-

## The Twist

When in position, take a deep breath in through the nose—hold the breath as you twist round and for the count — twist back, and exhale, relaxing for a few seconds before repeating.

## Slow Motion Firming

As you bend the knees in toward the chest, inhale deeply through the nose. Hold the breath as you extend the legs and exhale as the legs are lowered to the floor. Inhale as you reach forward and sit up—hold the breath while taking the legs and pulling the body forward, and exhale as the head relaxes over. Inhale gently as you roll back down the spine, exhaling when you are flat again, ready to repeat.